Your
YOGA
Workbook

Words and yoga instruction **Eve Boggenpoel**
Editor **Mary Comber**
Art editor **Kelly Flood**
Chief sub-editor **Sheila Reid**

Photography **Kirsty Owen @ Tapestry**
Hair & make-up **Nathalie Fournier @ Artistic Licence**
Model **Sarah Smith @ WModels**
Clothes **Ilu Destress Crop Top, £39; Ilu Destress Leggings, £52**
(http://ilufitwear.com)
Cover clothes **Model's own**
Retouching **Ricky Martin**

Publisher **Steven O'Hara**
Publishing Director **Dan Savage**
Marketing Manager **Charlotte Park**
Commercial Director **Nigel Hole**

D0493512

Printed by **William Gibbons and Sons, Wolverhampton**
ISBN 9781911639497

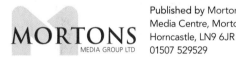

Published by Mortons Media Group Ltd,
Media Centre, Morton Way,
Horncastle, LN9 6JR
01507 529529

CONTENTS

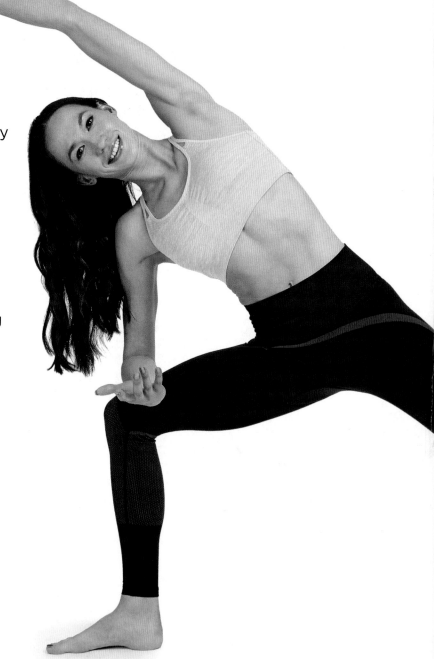

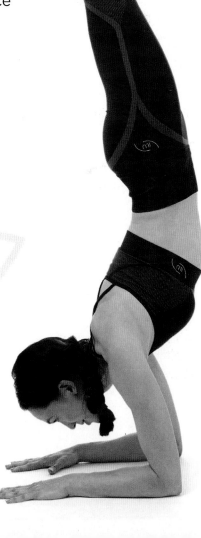

Twists

Backbends

Inversions

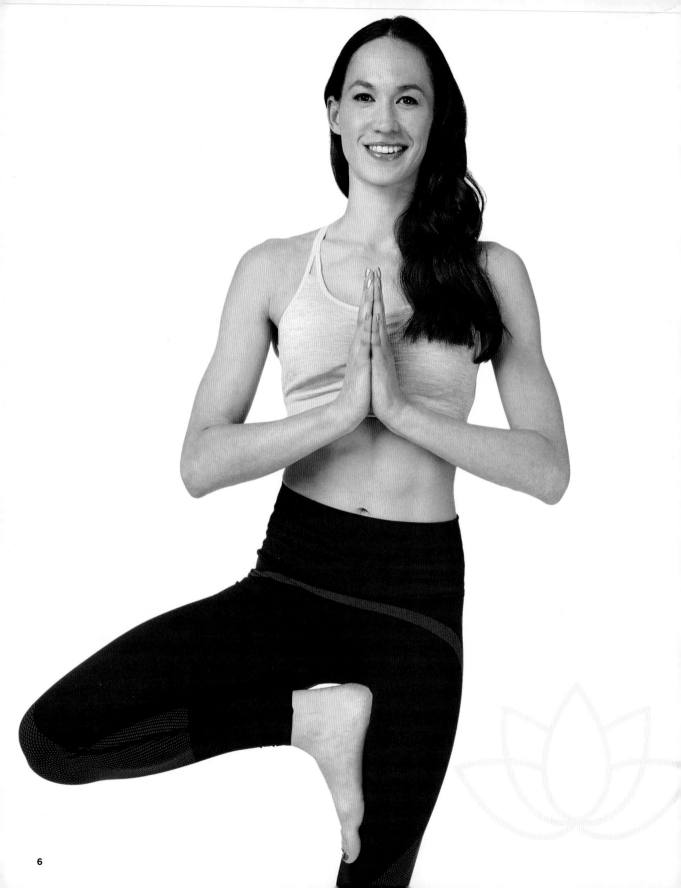

WELCOME

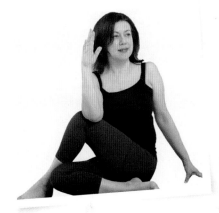

There comes a time in everyone's yoga journey when they want to take their experience that little bit deeper

Perhaps you don't have time to attend a class or maybe you've been doing the same class for a while and would like something different. Unfortunately, it's not always possible to go on an in-depth yoga retreat or to take a one-off intensive session on challenging poses.

If you'd like to progress your yoga practice, this book will help you. We've brought together 20 common postures and offer a mini masterclass in each one, to help you understand how the pose is constructed, and the ways in which it can benefit you. Each pose presents a particular challenge, whether it's maintaining an asymmetric balance or learning how to lift your body upwards in an inversion. Our step-by-step guide will give you the knowledge and technique you need to stay safe.

This book has come about in no small part as a result of my yoga teacher training at Triyoga in London (triyoga.co.uk). For two years, my tutors Mimi Kuo-Deemer and Jean Hall would workshop the poses we needed to learn for our training in a similar way to the method I've used here. We would study the pose in depth, looking at its benefits, contraindications, modifications and finer points of alignment. Most importantly, we would work on finding the fullest expression of the pose we could at that point in our experience. Each time we had a question, whether it was 'Should I rotate my arm inwards or outwards?' or 'What are the benefits of Headstand?' Mimi or Jean would say, 'Get on your mat and find out. See what it feels like in *your* body'.

I'm immensely grateful to Mimi and Jean for continually guiding me to trust my body, and I'd encourage you to do the same. We all have a unique anatomy and prior history of yoga, but it's only by learning from direct experience that something will truly make sense to you. My hope for this book is that it will help you become your own teacher. As you learn to trust your instinct, connect more deeply with the wisdom of your body and honour your limits, you'll become your own authority, and that will always be your best guide – both on and off your mat.

Namaste
Eve

ABOUT THE AUTHOR

Eve Boggenpoel has been practising yoga and meditation for 25 years. Self-taught initially, her formal yoga journey began with a German Iyengar teacher when she learnt to value the significance of good alignment, and went on to include vinyasa and yin styles with inspirational teachers Shiva Rea, Sarah Powers and Simon Low.

Eve is a qualified homeopath and health journalist, and author of several books, including *Yoga Calm, 10-Minute Mindfulness, Yoga Cures, 10-Minute AM/PM Yoga* and *Yoga, A Beginner's Guide.* In *Your Yoga Workbook*, Eve draws on her experience as a school teacher to bring together established ways to enhance your learning journey.

DEDICATION: *For Cary*

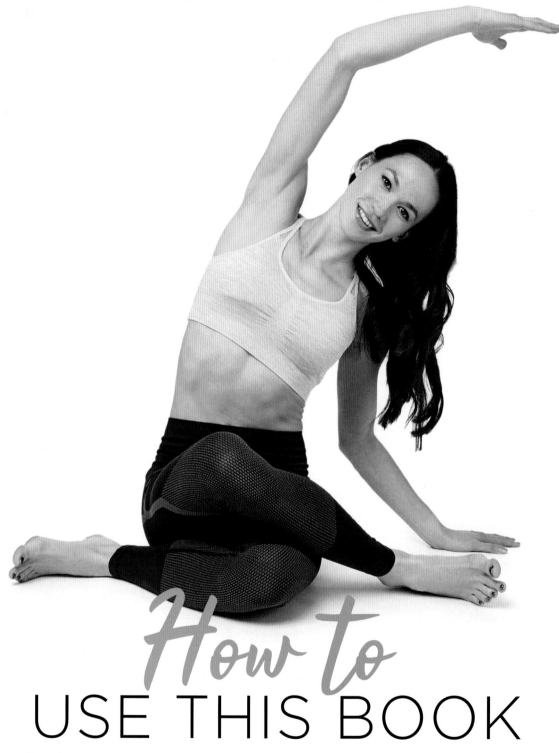

How to USE THIS BOOK

Can't wait to get started? Before you jump on your mat, read these guidelines to make sure you get the most out of your session

Yoga is a wonderful way to calm your senses, energise your body and focus your mind. All you need is time to practise the poses, and the more often you do, the greater the benefits. The ancient yogis spent years contemplating the interrelationship between body and mind, so the positioning of your body has specific effects. For instance, rooting through the base of your big and little toes in Tree (p56) doesn't just stabilise the posture, it also triggers a release of energy up through your body. And when your thumb (associated with

universal consciousness) and index finger (individuality) touch in Dancer (p68), you create an energetic circuit that connects you to your higher self, bringing a sense of calm. To enjoy these benefits fully, you need to deepen your understanding of the postures, fine-tune your alignment and learn to embody the postures more fully.

Read through the first section of this book to become familiar with a few key principles before moving on to the main poses. Then set aside around 30 minutes to workshop your chosen pose. You'll soon enjoy the benefits of a focused and in-depth practice.

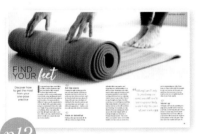

p12 YOUR YOGA WORKSHOP

One-pose practice is different to following a sequence of postures. Here we give you everything you need to know to make your session a success, from setting an intention to looking after your body, how to integrate your experience and the benefits of keeping a learning journal.

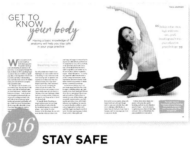

p16 STAY SAFE

A basic understanding of key anatomy principles will help to prevent injury and make sure you get the most out of your yoga session. Learn the moves that keep your spine in optimum health and discover the anatomical reasons why your knees need extra attention in bent leg poses.

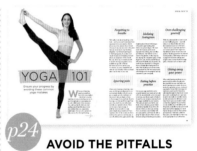

p24 AVOID THE PITFALLS

In *Yoga 101* we list the common mistakes to look out for. Discover the difference between good pain (the pose is gently stretching your muscles) and bad pain (it's time to stop), when to follow the advice of a teacher and when to be your own authority, and how not to sabotage your session.

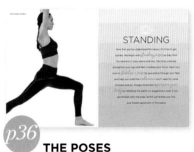

p36 THE POSES

Each chapter focuses on a different style of pose, such as standing, backbends or inversions. If you're fairly new to yoga, work through the chapter in order as the postures are presented in ascending level of difficulty, the initial poses giving you the skills needed for the more challenging ones.

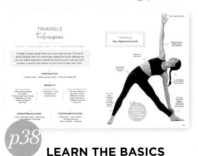

p38 LEARN THE BASICS

On the first two pages of each section, we introduce the pose you'll be workshopping. Learn what the pose's Sanskrit name means, discover its physical, mental and therapeutic benefits, understand the precautions and contraindications for practice and become familiar with the key alignment points.

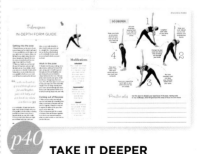

p40 TAKE IT DEEPER

On the second two pages of each section, our guidelines show you how to get into and out of the pose safely with suggestions for refining your alignment. We give modifications for inflexible bodies, and for those who're hypermobile or injured. We show you how to deepen the pose and give you space to record your experience.

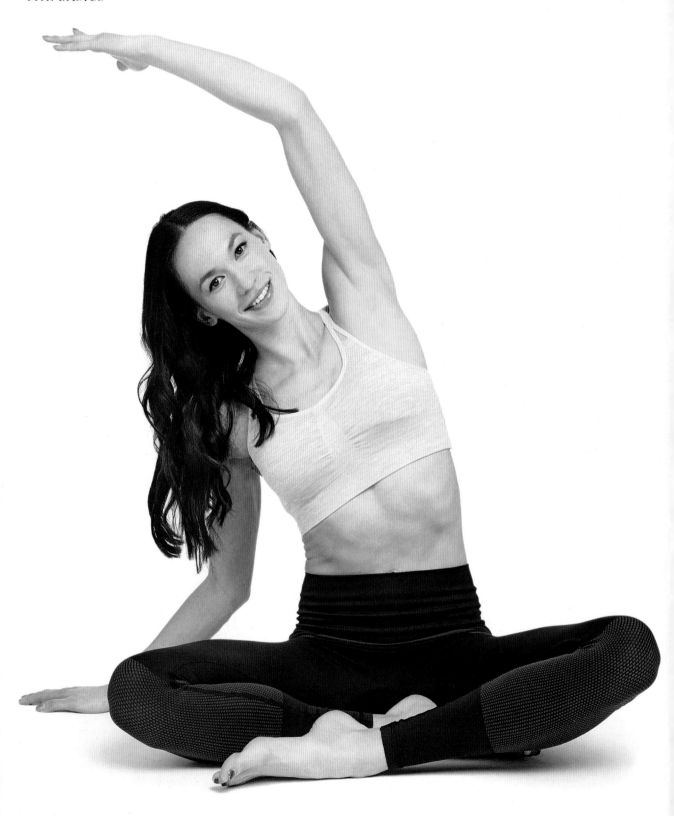

THE BASICS

Focusing on one pose at a time may be a new way of practising for you, so in this chapter we give you *lots of tips* on how to maximise your time on the mat. We show you how to protect your *spine and your knees*, which can be particularly vulnerable in yoga, and look at ways to *optimise your breathing*, not just to enhance your yoga practice but your general wellbeing as well. You'll also discover the common *yoga mistakes* to avoid and how to take you practice to the next level.

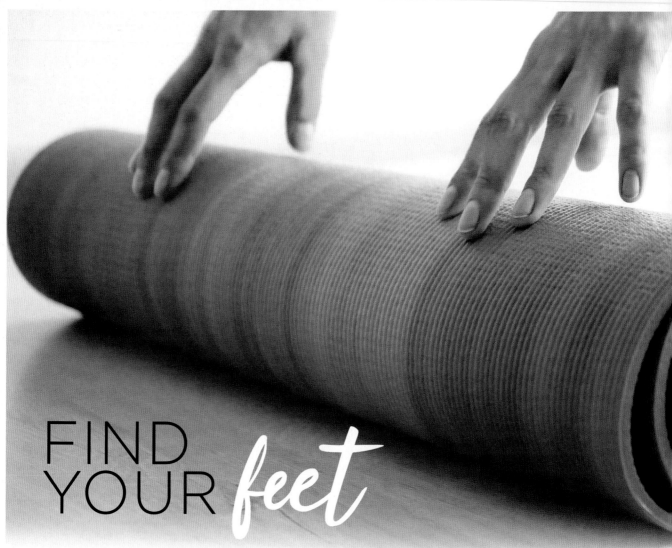

FIND
YOUR *feet*

Discover how to get the most from your one-pose practice

I n a general yoga class, you're likely to follow a series of postures that give your body a fully-rounded workout that stretches and strengthens all the major muscle groups in your body using standing and seated poses, forward and back bends, balances and inversions. One-pose practice is different. It gives you the opportunity to work in depth with a particular posture and get to understand it from the inside out. Think of it as a kind of masterclass or workshop, where you explore the pose from all angles and make it your own. Before you start, read the following advice to make sure you get the most out of your practice.

Set the scene

Creating the right environment for your one-pose practice will help you maximise your time on the mat. Set aside some time when you know won't be disturbed and turn your phone off. Along with your mat, extra layers of clothing for the relaxation section and any props, keep a pen and paper – or a dedicated yoga journal – handy, so you can make any notes about your session.

Have an intention

Having a clear goal can make all the difference between simply feeling

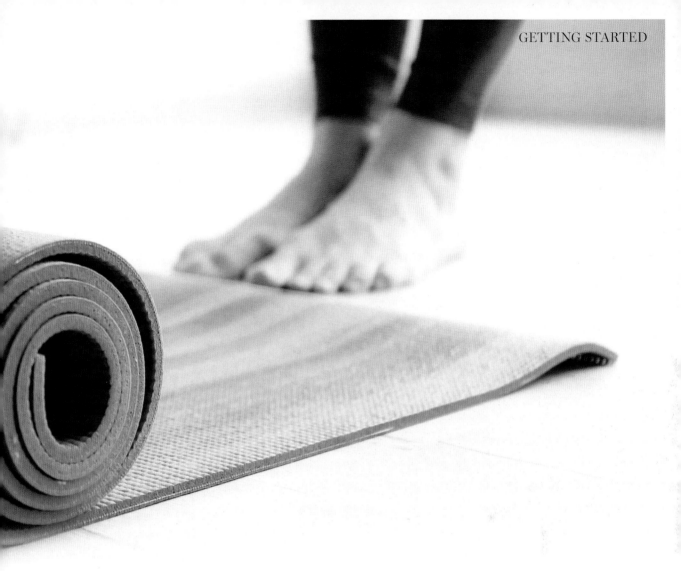

refreshed after your practice and deepening your understanding of, or skill in, a pose. Sometimes you might want to make a general intention, such as staying connected to your breath, working with closed eyes or exploring what it means to you to direct lines of energy through your body. On other occasions, try committing to something that relates directly to the posture you want to work on as this will accelerate your learning. For example, you may decide to focus on rotating your chest open in Revolved triangle (p86), or rooting through your forearms in Forearm balance (p122). This is also where your practice notes can be really helpful. So if one week you notice that

66 Although you'll only be practising one move, you still need to warm up your body, so don't skip this part of your session 99

you're compressing one side of your torso, in Prayer twist (p82) for example, in your next session on that pose, you could have the intention to learn as much as you can on lengthening both sides of your body equally.

Warm up

Although you'll only be practising one yoga move, you still need to warm up your body, so don't skip this part of your session. In some ways, it's even more important than if you're at a class, as your teacher will structure the sequence so the postures in the early part of the class warm the muscles and open the joints you'll need for the more complex poses at the end of the class. For each posture in this book we've included three poses from the Warm-up section (p30) that specifically target the parts of the body you'll be using. As you work your way through the poses and build an embodied experience of them, feel free to use poses from the main part of the book to prepare your body for the pose you are practising in that session. For example, Dancer pose (p68) needs strong balance and open hips, so you could spend a few moments in Tree pose (p56), and opening your groin in Wide-legged standing forward fold (p42), before devoting the remainder of your session to working on Dancer.

First things first

The book is structured so that each chapter begins with a simpler pose and works up to more challenging postures. For this reason, it's a good idea to work through each chapter sequentially. Gaining a solid, embodied foundation in the early poses will make the following ones easier to achieve. Similarly, work through the poses in the order presented in the chapter. Becoming familiar with the key alignment points will give you a good grounding in the essential areas you need to know before you work on fine-tuning the pose.

Choose wisely

You may already know the poses you wish to focus on, and if you've been practising yoga for a year or two, feel free to choose the poses you most want to improve. However, remember to mix up your practice, so you don't create any imbalances in your body. If you work on a backbend one session, do a forward bend the next or, if you spend a few days working on challenging inversions, balance this with restful seated or supine poses before going back to the more demanding poses. If you'd like to take a more structured approach, you could simply work your way through the book, choosing the first standing pose one week, the first balance the next, the first twist the week after and so on. As you progress, listen to your body and follow what it needs – it is, after all, your best teacher.

Look after your body

Your body is continually in flux. Along with changes due to ageing, fluctuations in your hormones during your menstrual cycle make you more flexible on some days than others, while on other occasions, for no particular reason, a posture that felt easy the day before may feel more challenging today. For each pose, we've included the major precautions and

> **❝** *Don't create imbalances in your body. If you work a backbend one session, do a forward bend the next* **❞**

contraindications for practice. If you have any of the conditions listed in the contraindications, speak to your GP before practising them or work on the pose with a suitably qualified yoga teacher. Milder conditions are listed under the precautions, and if you turn to the modifications section of the chapter, you'll find ways to adapt your practice accordingly. Most of all, listen to your body. Don't push it beyond its limits, but work on opening to a pose, gradually and sustainably over time.

Integrate your experience

Although you've only worked on one pose, don't be tempted to skip the relaxation pose at the end of your session. This is the time when your body will absorb the benefits of the pose, and give you the opportunity to reflect on and mentally integrate what you've learnt. It also means you won't rush headlong into your day and undo all the good you've created in your practice. Following the guidelines for Savasana (p35), and Legs up the wall (p34), ensure you're completely comfortable, making any minor adjustments you

need. You might want to play some relaxing music, place an eyebag over your eyes, or a bolster crosswise beneath your knees. Spend between five and 10 minutes in the pose, longer if you have the time. Not only will it allow your muscles to relax and heartbeat return to normal, it will also deeply nourish your nervous system, and leave you feeling refreshed for the next phase of your day.

Your learning journal

Keeping a note of your experiences while you practise is one of the best ways to maximise your learning – on all levels. Being in a mindful space will help you tune in more deeply to your body, and recording what you found challenging, what felt good and what you'd like to focus on in the future will broaden your understanding of the pose. Sometimes the changes you notice will feel wonderful – you'll experience a sense of inner strength, your body will feel in harmony with itself – like a finely tuned instrument – or you'll experience an inexplicable rush of energy.

At other times, you may feel nothing new or positive is happening and just feel irritated, frustrated or even sad. As well as challenging your body, yoga can bring up a range of emotions – if this happens to you, be kind to yourself and patient, and trust that your body knows what it is doing. If you have the time, ask your body what it most needs, and then create the space in your life to give that to yourself. Whatever comes up in your practice, make a note of it in your journal, being as detailed as feels comfortable for you, and use it as a treasure trove of information to learn from.

GET TO KNOW *your body*

Having a basic knowledge of anatomy will help you stay safe in your yoga practice

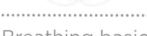

When you start to work in more depth on individual yoga poses it's useful to build up your understanding of anatomy at the same time. As you progress through this book, it's likely you'll be spending longer in postures than you would in a regular yoga class, so it's important to know how to protect your body. Understanding how your body works can also be helpful when you're not sure how to progress with a particular pose.

We will begin with the breath, as it's so central to yoga. Not only does it help create a calm state of mind and make you more body aware – which in itself helps prevent injury – it also fuels the more energetic postures and tells you when you're working too hard. Next, we'll look at how to keep your spine healthy and protected, and finally, we'll give a brief overview of the knee joint, which is especially vulnerable in yoga. If you bear these points in mind as you practise, we're sure you'll have a safe and enjoyable experience in this next stage of your yoga journey.

Breathing basics

You will probably have heard of your diaphragm, the main muscle involved in breathing. It comes from the Greek word meaning 'wall' or 'partition', and separates your chest cavity from your abdominal cavity. It's a large dome-shaped muscle that, when contracted, moves downwards, increasing the volume of your chest cavity. This results in a drop in air pressure in your lungs, which causes air to be drawn in. Likewise, when your diaphragm relaxes back to its resting position, it decreases the space in your lungs and air is forced out of your body.

We usually think of breathing as simply taking oxygen into our lungs and breathing out carbon dioxide, but breathing happens in two distinct phases – one external, the other internal. In the first phase, the one we're more familiar with, air is drawn into your lungs and oxygen is removed by the tiny air sacs called alveoli, and from here it's transported to every cell in your body. At the same time, the alveoli remove toxic carbon dioxide from the blood, which is expelled as you breathe out. In the second phase, internal respiration, oxygen – along with glucose – is used by tiny organelles called mitochondria to produce energy for movement, repair, reproduction and waste disposal, while carbon dioxide, a by-product of cellular activity, is returned to your lungs.

Several factors influence how well your lungs expand and, therefore, draw in oxygen, including posture, age, tight muscles, stress, heart health and illnesses where there is narrowing of the airways, such as in asthma. While we have no control over some of these factors, yoga can greatly improve posture, ease tight muscles and reduce stress, all of which influence your breathing. For example, to improve shoulder mobility try poses such as Eagle (p60), Cow face (p31) and Wide-legged standing forward fold (p42). For chest-opening poses, include Camel (p100), Cobra (p96) and

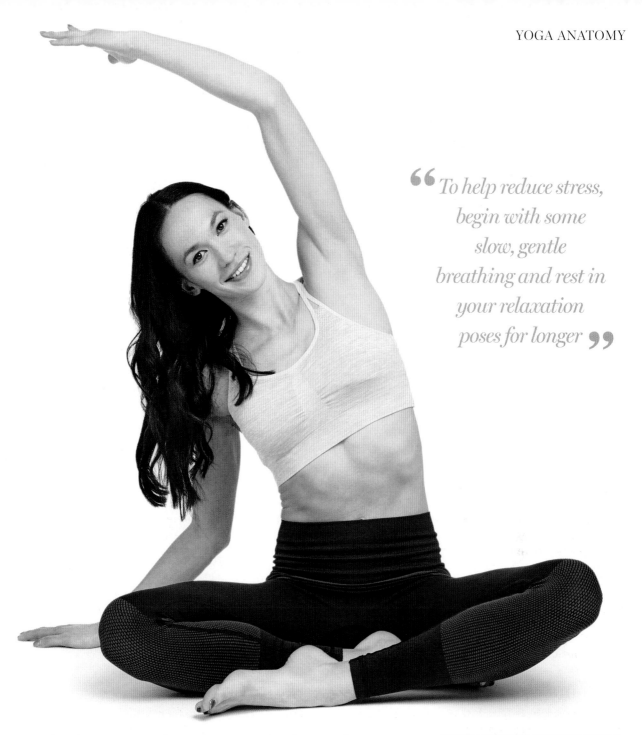

To help reduce stress, begin with some slow, gentle breathing and rest in your relaxation poses for longer

Bow (p104) in your practice, along with Seated side bend (p30)and Triangle (p38) to open your side ribs. You could also try placing a rolled blanket or bolster beneath the back of your heart in Savasana (p35) to encourage your chest to open more deeply.

To help reduce stress, begin your practice with some slow, gentle breathing, and rest in your relaxation poses for longer – up to 20 minutes. Lengthening your exhale will also help calm your mind, as this activates the parasympathetic nervous system.

For more ways to incorporate stress-busting breathing techniques into your everyday life, see p20-23.

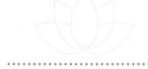

Save your spine

Your spine works hard and with a little knowledge you can help it do its job to the best of its ability. As well as bearing the weight of your upper body, your spine absorbs shock, provides stability and does the vitally important job of protecting your spinal cord. It also allows you to bend your torso in a wide variety of ways – flexion (forwards), extension (backwards), hyperextension (backwards beyond the normal range of movement), lateral flexion (sideways) and rotation. The range of movement in your spine depends on several factors – age, anatomy, genetics, injury history, time of day and lifestyle factors such as occupation, exercise habits, diet and posture – only some of which you have control over.

Despite this, yoga can help maintain and, indeed, improve your range of movement. As your muscles are more elastic when warm, it's a good idea to do a combination of gentle poses that take your spine through all its planes of movement – try Cat/Cow, Seated twist and Seated side bend (all p30) – before progressing onto postures where your spine is strongly flexed or extended. Encouraging length in your spine with poses such as Downward dog (p110), will also help its ability to flex, extend and rotate.

But a healthy spine isn't just about flexibility – strength and stability are important too. Remember that your core muscles play an important part in maintaining the stability of your spine – weak transversus abdominis, rectus

Remember your core muscles play an important part in maintaining the stability of your spine

abdominis or oblique muscles can lead to lumbar spine injury. Warm-up poses in this book to help develop core strength include Boat, Bicycle twist and Plank (all p33).

The health of your spine is also dependent on well-hydrated intervertebral discs. The fibrocartilage discs that separate the bones of your spine and provide its shock-absorbing properties lose around two per cent of their water content over the course of a day but, fortunately, yoga can help replenish this. When you move your vertebrae, the compression and release of the discs creates a kind of hydraulic pumping action that attracts fluid back into the area. For this reason, yoga moves such as Cat/Cow (p30), or sequences such as sun salutations, with their repeated spinal flexion and extension movements, are ideal for rehydrating your discs.

Protect your knees

Your knee is an amazing joint that carries your entire bodyweight at the same time as enabling the flexion and extension needed for walking, running, sitting, climbing and going up and down stairs. And when it comes to your yoga practice, it can be particularly vulnerable.

Unlike your hip joint, where the ball of your femur (thigh bone) sits deep within the socket of your pelvis, the bones of your knee joint don't provide much stability – the two rounded 'knuckles' at the lower end of your femur simply rest on the relatively flat surface of your tibia (shin bone). The extra support that

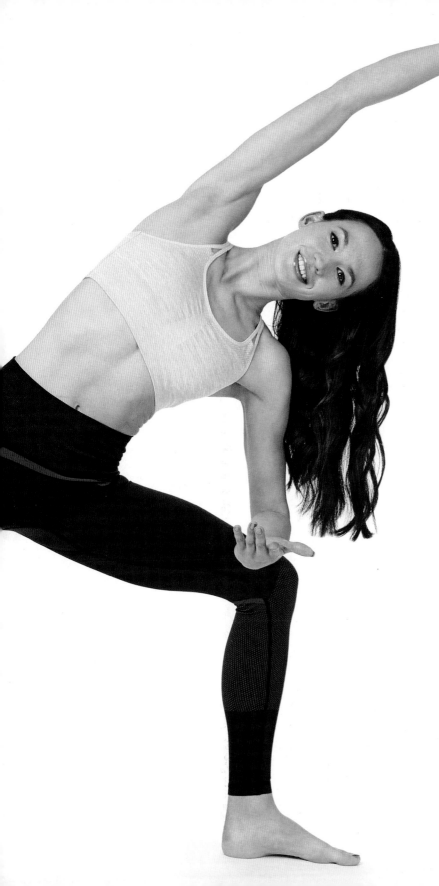

is needed is provided by soft tissue – cartilage and ligaments (which prevent your knee from displacing forwards, backwards and sideways) and the tendons of your quadriceps and hamstrings.

Muscle strength is enhanced by load bearing, therefore standing asanas, such as Warrior I (p46) where your quads contract to support your body's weight, will help strengthen them. Contracting your quads to raise the weight of your legs, as in Boat (p33), will also help build strength.

Stretching the muscles surrounding your knee will also help maintain its health. Tight quads can lead to knee pain and instability, increasing the risk of falls and premature wear and tear. If your quads are tight, spend time on poses that take your knee into flexion (Dancer, p68) or that lengthen your hip flexors (Crescent moon, p32 and Bow, p104). It's also important that the individual muscles of your quadriceps are balanced (your quads are made up of four different muscles) This will help reduce the chance of the patella (knee cap) misaligning, which could lead to wear and tear, knee pain and eventually arthritis. For optimum safety in yoga, check that your knee is aligned over your middle toe, especially when in bent leg postures such as Warrior I (p46).

Finally, it's not just how you use your knees in yoga that impacts on their health, your hips play a big part too, so working mindfully with asanas to gently encourage external rotation at the hip will also support knee health. If your hips are tight, regularly include Reclining twist (p78) in your practice to help prevent strained ligaments, tendonitis and maltracking of your patella and even a meniscus tear.

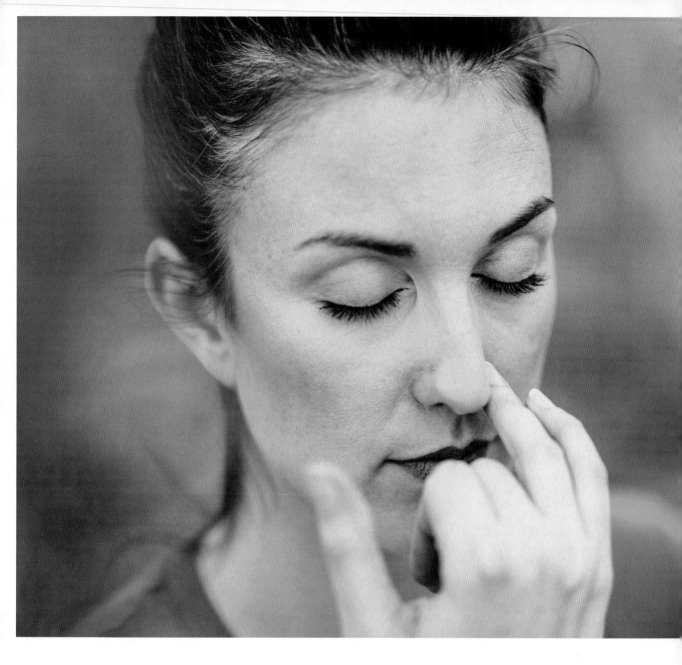

BE A BETTER
breather

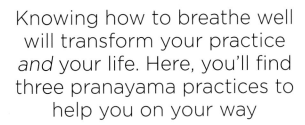

Knowing how to breathe well will transform your practice *and* your life. Here, you'll find three pranayama practices to help you on your way

One of the reasons your breath is so important is that it connects you to the present moment. When you're on your mat, instead of practising with a racing mind preoccupied with unfinished jobs or plans for later in the day, if you attune to your breath you strengthen your focus and become more sensitive to the physical sensations and energy moving through your body. Your perspective shifts and you see more clearly what matters, you sense the nature of things. You see beauty all around you and feel more grounded and centred in yourself. If this sounds a little esoteric, take a moment to explore it for yourself. Close your eyes, let your breath become slower and deeper until you are softly breathing into the base of your abdomen. Be soft. Relax. Trust. When you open your eyes, what do you notice? Our relationship to our breath is an enormous subject, and many of us are only just scratching the surface of it.

What may be more familiar is the awareness that your breath is the bridge that connects your body and your mind. When we feel anxious our breathing is rushed and shallow, when we're relaxed it becomes slow and deep. Conversely, we can choose to calm a troubled mind by consciously slowing down our breath. With one of the definitions of yoga being 'yoke' or 'union' – a practice that brings mind and body together – it's little wonder that breath plays such a central role. Another definition, from the ancient sage Patanjali, describes yoga as a practice for 'calming the fluctuations of the mind'. And if you've ever practised mindfulness breathing techniques, you'll know the power of the breath for stilling a busy mind.

In yoga, working with the breath begins with pranayama – prana means energy or life force and ayama means to extend – and its purpose, initially, is to help you learn to direct your breath in a beneficial way. Some people refer to it as controlling the breath, but another way to think of it is liberating your breath. See right and over, for three pranayama practices you can do in conjunction with your one-pose practice or individually throughout your week when you want to experience their benefits. But as well as working with pranayama, it's a good

Balance your system

Nadi shodana balances the right and left sides of your body, so is perfect to use with balance poses.

■ Sit in a comfortable position and take a moment to centre yourself. Bring your right hand to your nose, and rest the tip of your thumb on the fleshy part of your right nostril while placing the tips of your index and middle fingers between your eyebrows. Curl your ring and little fingers under, and rest the inside of your ring finger on your left nostril.

■ Close your left nostril with your ring finger and exhale fully through your right nostril. Keeping your left nostril closed, inhale fully and slowly through your right nostril, then close it with your thumb, and release your ring finger to open your left nostril and exhale slowly. Pause, then inhale slowly through your left nostril. Close off this nostril with your ring finger, pause, and release your right nostril with your thumb, then exhale slowly and steadily through this nostril. This forms one round. Repeat, breathing slowly and mindfully for five minutes.

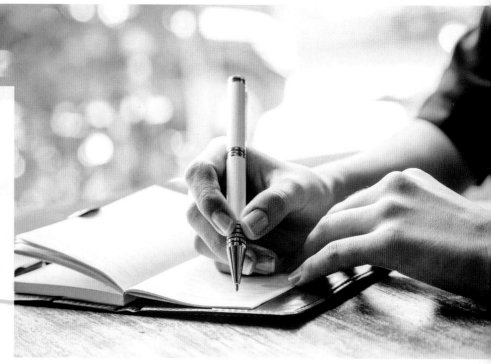

Get energised

Kapalabhati breathing energises your whole body very quickly. Do not practise it if you are pregnant, menstruating or after eating.

■ Sit in a comfortable position and connect to your breathing for a few moments to centre yourself. When ready, place your hands on your belly and draw your navel in and up as you exhale quickly through your nose. Don't consciously breathe in, but allow inhalation to happen naturally. Repeat this pattern four to eight times, noticing your belly move in and out like a bellows beneath your hands, and ending with an out-breath. This is one cycle.

■ Do another three or four cycles, gradually increasing the speed of your breath, so each exhalation lasts around one second. Take a few, deep abdominal breaths after each cycle to rest your lungs and diaphragm. As you become more experienced, you can build up to 15–30 breaths per cycle.

idea to become more aware of how you breathe in everyday life and learn how you can liberate your breath off as well as on your mat.

Keep a breathing journal

When we've spent years not really being conscious of our breath, keeping a breathing journal can be a useful way to understand how you breathe, and teach you how to breathe more fully. To begin, aim to check in with your breath at three different points during the day and make a note of your observations. Depending on what works best for you, either check in at the same time every day, for example, on waking, just after you eat your lunch and on your journey home from work. Or, just commit to tuning in to your breath at three moments throughout the day. These could be completely random, or you may decide to work with a particular emotion, say stress, and observe your breathing pattern whenever you notice

stressful feelings beginning to arise.

As you record your observations, you'll soon begin to notice some patterns emerge – maybe you find you take shallow chest breaths when you feel anxious, or perhaps you hold your breath completely when you're concentrating at work. You may discover that you rarely fully inhale or you never really empty your lungs. Initially, try not to change your breathing pattern when you check in – just notice *how* you are breathing. As you become more familiar with how you breathe, it may prompt you to inquire further and ask yourself questions, such as, 'If I'm holding back my breath, what else am I holding back? My anger? My sadness? My right to express myself?'

Over the weeks, you'll build up an invaluable resource that you'll be able to use to help you to learn to breathe more fully and experience all the benefits that brings, from removing toxins from your system more thoroughly to leaving you feeling full of energy and vitality.

Fuel your practice

Ujjayi breathing is a great way to support your yoga practice. Ujjayi means victorious breath, and breathing in this way can help fuel your body, especially when you're working in depth with more challenging poses. If you're not familiar with the technique, practise ujjayi on its own a few times before using it in your one-pose yoga sessions.

■ Sit in a comfortable position, close your eyes and gradually deepen your breathing, inhaling to a count of three and exhaling to a count of six, allowing the pause period between breaths to lengthen naturally. Consciously release any tension as you exhale.

■ After a few minutes, let your breathing return to normal. Gently open your lips and this time breathe in and out through your mouth, making a soft, whispering 'haaa' sound as you do so. This action slightly closes your throat, which is the main physiological action of ujjayi breathing. After a few rounds, close your lips together, but still breathe in the same way, as if you were making the 'haaa' sound. Aim to keep the quality of your breathing very gentle, so the sound would only be audible to someone sitting close to you. Continue in this way for a few minutes then gently let it go, and softly open your eyes.

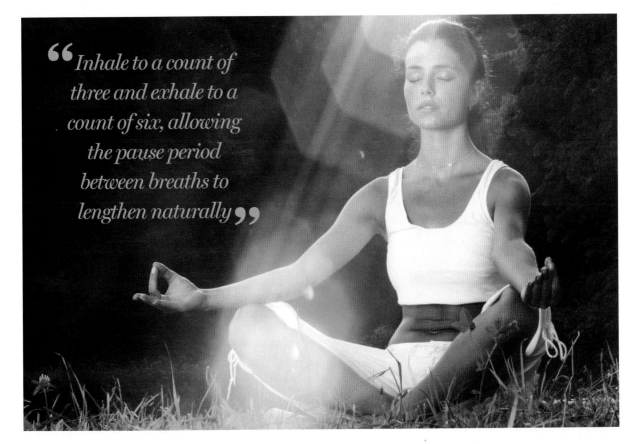

Inhale to a count of three and exhale to a count of six, allowing the pause period between breaths to lengthen naturally

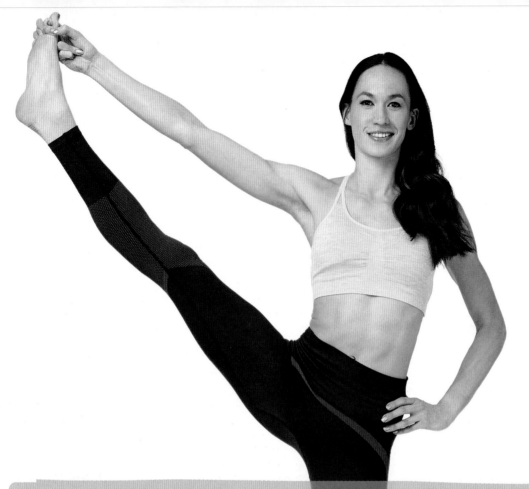

YOGA 101

Ensure your progress by avoiding these common yoga mistakes

When you're learning yoga by yourself you have to be extra vigilant – there's isn't a teacher watching over you, reminding you not to push through pain or encouraging you to work a little harder when necessary. You could say that it's when you start guiding yourself and listening to your own wisdom that your yoga journey really begins. Here are a few pointers to help you set off on the right footing.

Forgetting to breathe

We've talked a lot about breathing in this book – and by now you'll understand how important it is to your practice. But it's all too easy to be unaware of your breath when you're on your mat, even to the point that you momentarily stop breathing altogether. And it doesn't just happen in challenging poses, it can also occur simply because you're thinking too hard about your alignment. If this sounds like you, find a way to remind yourself to breathe during your practice. Use a meditation app with a Tibetan bell timer and set it to chime every 10 minutes, or source a beautiful card with the word 'breathe' written on it and place it at the front of your mat.

Idolising Instagram

Social media is littered with images of beautiful yogis bending their bodies into pretzel shapes. The more exotic the location and the more expensive the clothing, the more likes and followers. And while it can be a source of inspiration, it often traps us into playing the comparison game. If that happens to you, remind yourself that an influencer's flexibility may be genetic, the result of years of practise or a hangover from a classical dance background. So rather than looking up to someone else, stay grounded in your own yoga journey, acknowledge your own progress and stay connected to your own goals.

Over-challenging yourself

While it's understandable to want to work on more challenging poses – especially when you see them broken down into their constituent parts as in this book – learn to listen to your body and don't over-extend yourself. Don't neglect the foundations in favour of more advanced postures. Standing poses form the bedrock of your practice, so feel strong in the poses on pages 38-53, before working more complex twists, such as Revolved triangle (p86), or balances such as Dancer (p68).

Giving away your power

When you're learning anything new, you need to seek the advice of people who have travelled the same road before you, but it's important not to make others too much of an authority over you. Acclaimed yoga teacher Donna Fahri encourages her students to experiment for themselves with what feels right for their body. So next time you're wondering if your upper arm should be internally or externally rotated, try both and notice the difference in your body. Does it open your shoulder blades or draw them together? Do you feel less or more stability in your shoulder joint? What is its overall effect on the pose? You'll learn more by fully engaging your mind than by taking on someone else's opinion and experience. Their body is different from yours, and what's right for them may not be appropriate for you all the time.

Ignoring pain

When you're focusing on learning a new pose, or refining your alignment in one you're already familiar with, it's easy to get so caught up in the mechanics of the posture that you forget to listen to the messages from your body. If you're hearing a cue that says lift strongly from your chest, don't let your enthusiasm override your natural instincts. There are two types of pain in yoga. A mild but consistent ache is a sign you're lengthening a muscle and if you experience this it's fine to carry on, but a sudden, sharp pain is a warning sign, so ease off a little and try again another day.

Eating before practice

Get on your yoga mat before you've properly digested your meal and not only will it be uncomfortable to do twists and inversions, your blood supply will also be focused in your stomach, meaning there's less oxygen available for your muscles. That said, you need some fuel in your body, so have a banana, peanut butter sandwich or handful of nuts 30 to 60 minutes before you start your session. Once you become more familiar with one-pose practice, you'll soon be able to judge the right amount of time to leave between eating and starting your session.

7 ways
TO TAKE YOUR PRACTICE TO THE NEXT LEVEL

It takes time and energy to move on in your yoga journey,
but follow our tips and you'll soon reap the rewards

I f you feel your practice is not moving forwards, don't worry, it means you're ready to learn more. Commit to dedicating extra time and energy to your yoga journey and you'll soon reap the benefits. To get you started, here are a few ways to immerse yourself more fully in your practice. And remember, short regular sessions will be more beneficial than a long one less frequently, so aim to get on your mat at least three or four times a week.

1 Step out of your comfort zone

Practising poses you are familiar with and can do well feels good and lets you experience yoga's benefits, but if you remain in your comfort zone you won't challenge yourself to learn anything new. So if you've been avoiding challenging balances or demanding inversions, plan to include them in your practice. Start gradually and build up as your confidence increases. Likewise, if you know you have good flexibility

but your upper body strength is weak, spend more time on core Warm-ups (p30-33). Not only will you develop stronger abdominal muscles, poses such as Headstand and Forearm balance will also be much easier.

2 Teach a friend

Team up with a yoga buddy and teach each other the poses you'd most like to learn. The old adage that while you teach you learn is true when it comes to yoga. Use the key alignment points in this book as a reference and guide your partner through the pose. As you gain more experience, move on to the more advanced alignment cues in the 'Go deeper' guides. Teaching someone else encourages you to look closely at another body in the posture and instantly shows you the modifications they need to make in order to do the pose well. It also helps you internalise the alignment cues so you remember to do them when you practise the pose yourself.

3 Practise in front of a mirror

If you don't have a yoga buddy to work with you can also gain a lot from practising in front of a mirror. We often think our arms are perpendicular to the floor in Triangle (p38), for example, only to see in the mirror that our top arm is at an angle. Until you hone your proprioception skills (your unconscious perception of your body in space), observing your reflection can help you associate the exact position your body is in with how you experience it internally.

4 Take notes

Yoga teachers may have spent half a day learning how to teach a pose – and half a lifetime perfecting it in their own practice – so they have a lot of wisdom to pass on. They also know the common challenges students face in a pose and how to guide them skilfully to overcome them. Unfortunately, that gem you heard while trying not to topple over

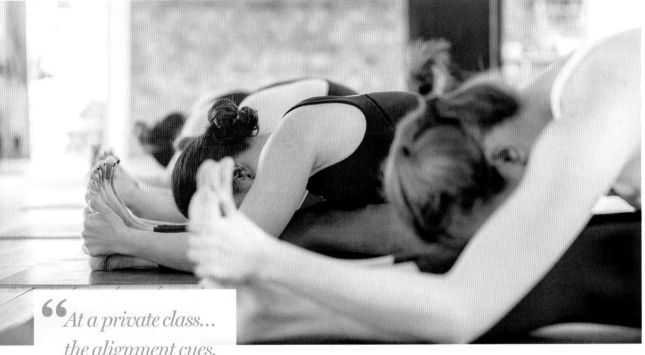

> **At a private class... the alignment cues, adjustments and feedback will be tailored to your ability, body type, injury history and interests**

in Eagle pose (p60) is often forgotten by the time you reach the changing room, let alone a week later when you're practising it at home. Take a notebook with you to class and jot down any comments that are pertinent to you, either before you get into the pose or while the teacher is still speaking, then refer to your notes during your yoga sessions at home. You'll soon see your practice growing in leaps and bounds.

5 Book a private lesson

If you feel you're stuck in your yoga journey, booking a one-off private lesson can show you how to improve your practice and provide you with a new direction. A private session will be tailored to your exact needs – not only can you ask the teacher what you want to work on, because you have 100 per cent of their attention, the alignment cues, adjustments and feedback will also be tailored to your ability, body type, injury history and interests. Book an appointment for a few weeks away, then each time you practise, make a note of anything you'd like to work on or questions you'd wish to ask.

6 Observe a class

Many schools of yoga require trainee teachers to spend several weeks observing classes being taught by experienced teachers. When there are 30 people in front of you all doing the same posture, you'll quickly see what good alignment looks like. You'll also notice what a student needs to do differently in order to bring a pose into balance. If you've built up a relationship with your teacher, ask if you could quietly sit at the back and observe one of their classes. Larger studios with bigger classes and/or teacher training programmes will be more familiar with having student observers sitting in, so you could try asking there if it's not possible at your local class.

7 Take the same class twice

Again, if you have a good relationship with your teacher, ask if they would mind if you record the class you're taking on your mobile, so you can practise it again at home. Explain that you're trying to deepen your practice, and you'd like the opportunity to work more consciously and consistently with the poses being taught. Don't worry about putting the teacher on the spot, sometimes, knowing that they're being recorded gives them the opportunity to settle into a more focused place in themselves and deliver the best lesson they can.

NEXT GENERATION *yoga props*

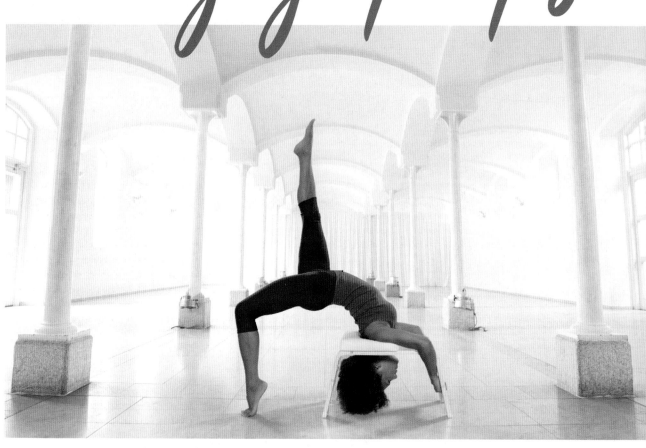

If you want to take your yoga practice a step further, try these two props

You're probably already familiar with the most common yoga props and how they can benefit you. Whether you need to extend the reach of your arms with a yoga strap, help maintain a neutral spine by sitting on a foam block, or release more deeply into Savasana by placing a bolster beneath your knees, most yoga studios will usually be able to accommodate you. Indeed, you're quite likely to have started to build a collection of your favourite props to assist your practice at home. Because of their multifunctional use, here are two more props we think are good investments when you want to progress your yoga practice.

PHOTOGRAPHY: YOGAMATTERS

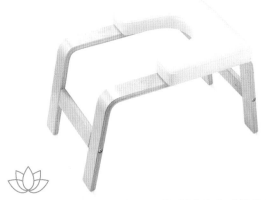

FEETUP HEADSTAND YOGA STOOL
£97.20; yogamatters.com

This stool is a great addition to your yoga kit. Made from birchwood and soft padded faux leather, it was designed by German yoga teacher Kilian Trenkle to remover the pressure from your head and neck while in Headstand. Your neck is vulnerable in inversions, but this stool prevents your shoulders from being compressed, and creates zero pressure on your cervical spin. It won't do the work for you, though, you're still going to need a strong core to rise up into the pose – perhaps more so given your legs and feet have further to lift than if you come into the pose from your mat - but it's a great support to anyone with a weak neck or shoulders. And you're likely to be able to remain in the pose longer, too, which is ideal as the longer you're in the posture the more benefits you experience.

How to use:

■ Rest the back edge of the stool against a wall. Snuggle your head into the gap, rest your shoulders on the padded cushion and your hands on the wooden supports. Let your neck release and soften. Raise your hips up and walk your feet towards your hands so you are in a deeply inverted 'V' shape. Push into your hands and raise your hips so they are over your shoulders. If you have a strong core, keep both legs straight and lift them overhead, so your feet are directly over your pelvis. Alternatively, bend one knee at a time to bring your knees into your chest in an inverted tuck position. Slowly and with control, raise both your legs to vertical. Remain in the pose for as long as you feel comfortable, then lower on an exhale, with control.
■ If you're confident in Headstand the FeetUp stool can help you progress further. Experiment with inverted splits – separating your legs forwards and backwards or out to the sides – wrap your legs around each other, as in eagle pose, bring the soles of the feet together, knees out to the sides, lower into a tuck and twist your torso to each side. You can also use the stool to work with arm balances, inverted backbends and even incorporate Headstands into a Sun salute. Each stool comes with a comprehensive guide.

DHARMA MITTRA SPECIAL EDITION CLASSIC YOGA WHEEL77
£65; yogamatters.com

Originally created by Dharma Yoga founder Sri Dharma Mittra and his son Yogi Varuna, dharma wheels are ideal for opening your chest, back, shoulders and hip flexors. Most are around 33cm in diameter and 13cm wide, so there's enough support for your spine, and the padded surround cushions your vertebrae for a comfortable stretch. There are a myriad ways to use a yoga wheel, but here are a few to get you started.

How to use:

■ **Chest opener:** Place the yoga wheel lengthways down the centre of your mat and lie back over it with the highest point in the centre of your mid-back. Rest your arms out to the side and release your neck backwards, allowing the curve of the wheel to open your back naturally.
■ **Back opener:** Sit on your mat with your legs straight in front of you. Place the wheel under your calf muscles and grasp its edges with your hands. Inhale as you lengthen your spine out of your waist, then as you exhale fold forwards, leading with your chest, using the wheel to pull you deeper.
■ **Shoulder stretch:** From Puppy dog pose (p31), take your knees further apart, and rest your hands on the wheel in front of you. Extend through your crown, so your neck is in line with your spine, then slowly roll the wheel forwards as you lower your chest towards the ground. Take a few deep breaths then exhale to return to the starting position.
■ **Hip flexor stretch:** From a Warrior I stance (p46), rest your back shin on the wheel. This will challenge your balance and strengthen your front thigh. Remember to swap sides.

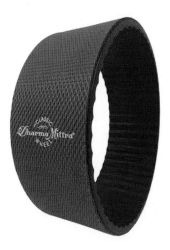

The WARM-UP

Prepare the body parts you'll be using for your one-pose practice, so you don't get injured

Moves for your SPINE

SEATED TWIST

Sit with crossed legs, heels aligned with your pubic bone, and place your left hand on the floor behind your left buttock, fingers pointing backwards. Rest your right palm on the outside of your right knee. Inhale as you root through your sitting bones to lift your spine out of your pelvis. On an exhale, rotate your spine to the left, moving in a spiral, first from your waist, then upper body. Inhale, lengthen through the crown of your head, exhale further into the twist. Draw your kidney area forwards and abdomen towards your navel. Inhale one last time, exhale, release further into the twist, turning to look over your left shoulder if comfortable for your neck. Inhale back to centre and repeat on the other side.

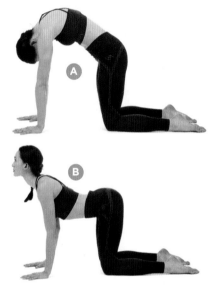

CAT/COW

From all-fours, inhale, then, as you exhale, root through the base of your index fingers and thumbs and the tops of your toes as you release your head and tailbone to the floor and lift your spine towards the ceiling into Cat (A). On your next inhale, tilt your tailbone up and release your spine down into a gentle backbend. Draw your shoulders down your back, take your chest forwards and up and gently raise your head into Cow (B). Continue alternating between Cat and Cow, instigating the movement from your pelvis and following the natural pattern of your breath. Move vertebra by vertebra in a slow and fluid way.

BENEFITS
✦ Extends and flexes your spine ✦ Massages your spinal discs

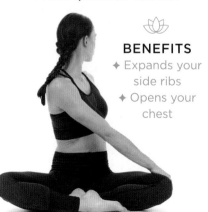

BENEFITS
✦ Expands your side ribs
✦ Opens your chest

SEATED SIDE BEND

Sit with crossed legs, heels aligned with your pubic bone, your right hand resting on the floor beside your right hip. Inhale and sweep your left arm in an arc overhead. Exhale. Inhale, root through your left sitting bone, lifting out of your waist. As you exhale, draw your left hand further over to the right, keeping your body on the same plane. Slide your right hand out to the side to rest on your forearm. Inhale, root down and lengthen, exhale and fold further to the right. Take a deep breath and come back to centre. Exhale, lower your left arm and repeat on the other side.

BENEFITS
✦ Mobilises your spine
✦ Creates space between vertebrae

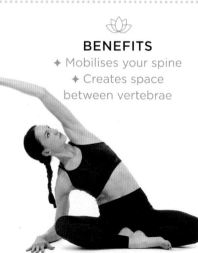

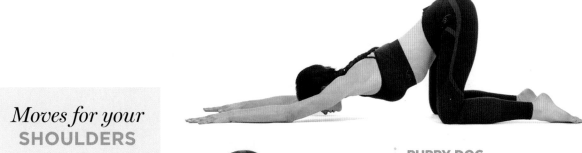

Moves for your SHOULDERS

THREAD THE NEEDLE

From Puppy dog (pictured, top), with your shoulders over your wrists and hips over your knees, inhale and raise your right arm out to the side. On an exhale, slide your right arm beneath your torso, palm facing up, extending your hand under your left arm and out to the side. Rest your head on the floor looking to your left side. Then take your left hand forwards a few inches and press into the floor to lift your left shoulder and deepen the twist. Exhale to release and repeat on the other side.

BENEFITS

✦ Opens your upper and outer shoulder muscles
✦ Releases tension between your shoulder blades

PUPPY DOG

From all-fours, with your shoulders over your wrists and hips over your knees, lie your toes flat on the floor and walk your hands forwards a hand's-length or two. Inhale, then exhale and root through your hands as you take your hips back slightly to lengthen your spine. Walk your hands forwards a few inches more, if needed, to keep your thighs vertical, then, with your arms remaining active and fingers spread, lower your head to the floor or a folded blanket. Relax your neck and take five deep breaths into your back body. To come out, exhale and walk your hands back in, come back up to kneeling and rest for a moment or two.

BENEFITS

✦ Opens your shoulders
✦ Stretches your spine

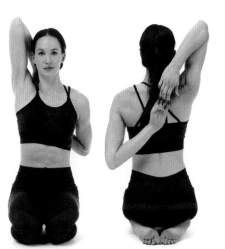

COW FACE POSE

From keeling, toes touching and ankles out to the side, inhale and raise your right arm out to the side at shoulder height. Rotate your palm to face the ceiling, then continue raising your arm until your upper arm is close to your ear. As you exhale, fold your forearm to rest your palm on the centre of your upper back, elbow pointing up. Inhale and raise your left arm out to the side, about 45 degrees. Turn your palm to face the back of the room, then bend your elbow and place the back of your hand between your shoulder blades, and take hold of the fingertips of your right hand. Take three to five deep breaths into your belly, rooting through your sitting bones to keep your spine long and your chest open. Release on an exhale and repeat on the other side.

BENEFITS

✦ Stretches your shoulders
✦ Releases the muscles in your upper arm

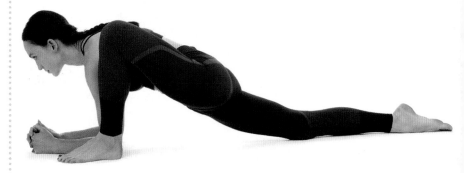

Moves for your HIPS

CRESCENT MOON

From standing, fold forwards and slide your left leg back, lowering onto your knee and the top of your left foot. Spread the toes of your right foot, root through your big and little toes and lift your inner arch. Inhale as you take your arms overhead, release your hips towards the floor as you exhale. Draw your belly button towards your spine, tuck your tailbone under and square your hips to give your left hip flexor a good stretch. Be in the pose for five to 10 breaths, breathing smoothly into your belly. To come out, exhale and lower your hands either side of your front foot. Step forwards with your back foot and return to standing, then repeat on the other side.

LIZARD

From crescent moon, hands either side of your front foot, raise your left hand as you heel/toe your foot towards the edge of your mat, then lower again. Raise your back knee and rest the front of your foot on the mat. Check that your front knee is directly above your ankle, hug it into the mid-line and ground through the base of your big and little toes. Walk your hands slightly forwards as you release your hips forwards and down, and extend your heart forwards to lengthen your spine while simultaneously drawing your shoulders down your back. Lightly draw your navel to your spine. If comfortable, lower onto your forearms, and take up to for five deep breaths. Press your hands into the mat to come back up, then repeat on the other side.

BENEFITS
✦ Opens your hips and groin ✦ Releases tight hip flexors

RECLINING HAND TO TOE POSE

Lie on your back and hug your right knee in to your chest. Grasp your right foot or calf with your right hand and on an inhale, straighten your leg in the air. Exhale as you rotate your hip outwards and lower your leg to the side. If necessary, use your left hand to keep your left hip on the floor, otherwise, extend your left arm out to the side. Take five to 10 deep breaths, inhale to bring your leg back to centre and exhale to gently lower. Repeat on the other side.

BENEFITS
✦ Opens your hips and groin
✦ Stretches your hamstrings

BENEFITS
✦ Stretches your hip flexors
✦ Strengthens your quadriceps

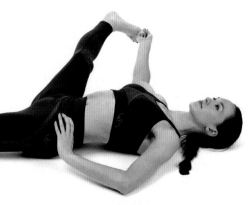

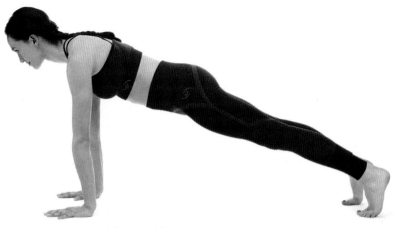

Moves to STRENGTHEN your CORE

PLANK

Start on all-fours with your hands shoulder-width apart, directly beneath your shoulders. Spread your fingers, root through the base of your thumbs and index fingers and straighten your elbows without locking them. Step your feet back, resting on the balls of your feet, and straighten your legs to create a diagonal line from your heels to your crown. Tuck in your chin to maintain length in the back of your neck. Draw your navel to your spine and spread your shoulder blades apart. Breathe evenly for five to 10 breaths, then lower on an exhale. Build up to one minute.

BENEFITS
✦ Strengthens your core, arms and upper body

BOAT

Sit on your mat, bend your knees, raise your feet off the floor and grasp the back of your thighs. Draw your navel to your spine and lean back to balance on your sitting bones. Take a few breaths, then raise your legs until your shins are parallel to the floor. If you're comfortable, extend your arms and hold them parallel to the floor. Take another few breaths, and, if balanced, straighten your legs to go into a 'V' shape. Draw your shoulder blades down your spine and keep your abdominals engaged, but your feet relaxed. Take up to five breaths, before releasing on an exhale.

BENEFITS
✦ Strengthens your abdominals and back muscles

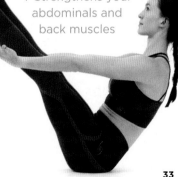

BICYCLE TWISTS

Lie on your back and rest your hands behind your head. Bend your knees to 90 degrees and raise over your hips. Inhale and draw your right elbow to your left knee, bringing your left knee in to meet it. Simultaneously straighten your right leg, close to, but not touching, the floor (A). Exhale and, twisting your torso, repeat the move on the other side, left elbow to right knee (B). Draw your navel to your spine throughout, pressing your lower back to the floor. Moving slowly and with control, repeat 20 times (10 on each leg), inhaling to move to the left, exhaling to move to the right.

BENEFITS
✦ Strengthens your upper and lower abdominals

The COOL DOWN

Relaxing your body after your one-pose practice will help you absorb the benefits of the pose

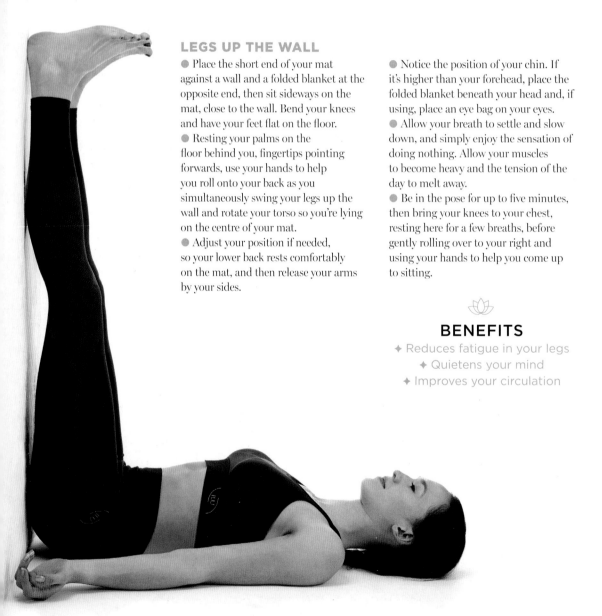

LEGS UP THE WALL

● Place the short end of your mat against a wall and a folded blanket at the opposite end, then sit sideways on the mat, close to the wall. Bend your knees and have your feet flat on the floor.

● Resting your palms on the floor behind you, fingertips pointing forwards, use your hands to help you roll onto your back as you simultaneously swing your legs up the wall and rotate your torso so you're lying on the centre of your mat.

● Adjust your position if needed, so your lower back rests comfortably on the mat, and then release your arms by your sides.

● Notice the position of your chin. If it's higher than your forehead, place the folded blanket beneath your head and, if using, place an eye bag on your eyes.

● Allow your breath to settle and slow down, and simply enjoy the sensation of doing nothing. Allow your muscles to become heavy and the tension of the day to melt away.

● Be in the pose for up to five minutes, then bring your knees to your chest, resting here for a few breaths, before gently rolling over to your right and using your hands to help you come up to sitting.

BENEFITS

✦ Reduces fatigue in your legs
✦ Quietens your mind
✦ Improves your circulation

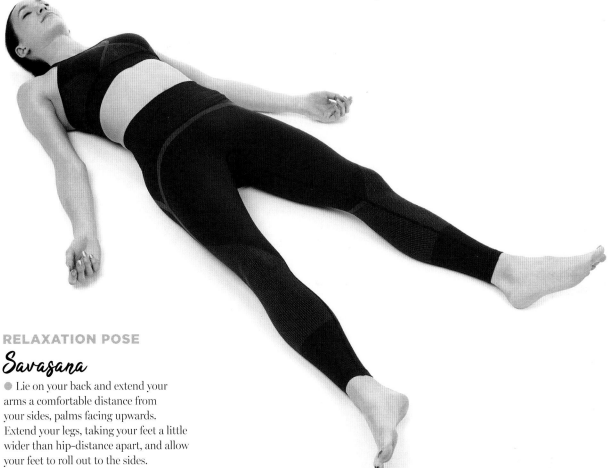

RELAXATION POSE
Savasana

 Lie on your back and extend your arms a comfortable distance from your sides, palms facing upwards. Extend your legs, taking your feet a little wider than hip-distance apart, and allow your feet to roll out to the sides.

● Wriggle your torso a little, to snuggle your body into the floor then, checking that your arms and legs are symmetrical, rest your head on the centre of the back of your skull. Gently close your eyes.

● Breathe softly and evenly into your belly, letting your eyelids be heavy, your jaw soft and your belly relaxed. In your one-pose practice, you may have worked in a more focused way than usual, so allow any tension built up in your session to release on each exhalation.

● Rest for a few moments, then let your breath become a little slower and deeper, making your out-breath slightly longer than your in-breath.

● Spend some time reflecting on the pose you have focused on today, how did your body feel before you practised? How does it feel now? What aspects of the pose felt challenging? What felt good? What would you like to do differently next time?

● Let your breath return to normal, and rest in the pose for five to 10 minutes, feeling a gentle sense of expansion as you inhale, and softening as you exhale.

● To come out of the pose, wriggle your fingers and toes. Slide your arms out to the sides and overhead, and gently stretch your body from your feet to your fingertips. Slowly bring your knees to your chest, roll over to your right side and rest for few moments, then use your left hand to help you come up to sitting.

BENEFITS
✦ Calms your mind
✦ Reduces fatigue
✦ Rejuvenates
✦ Balances your mind, body and spirit

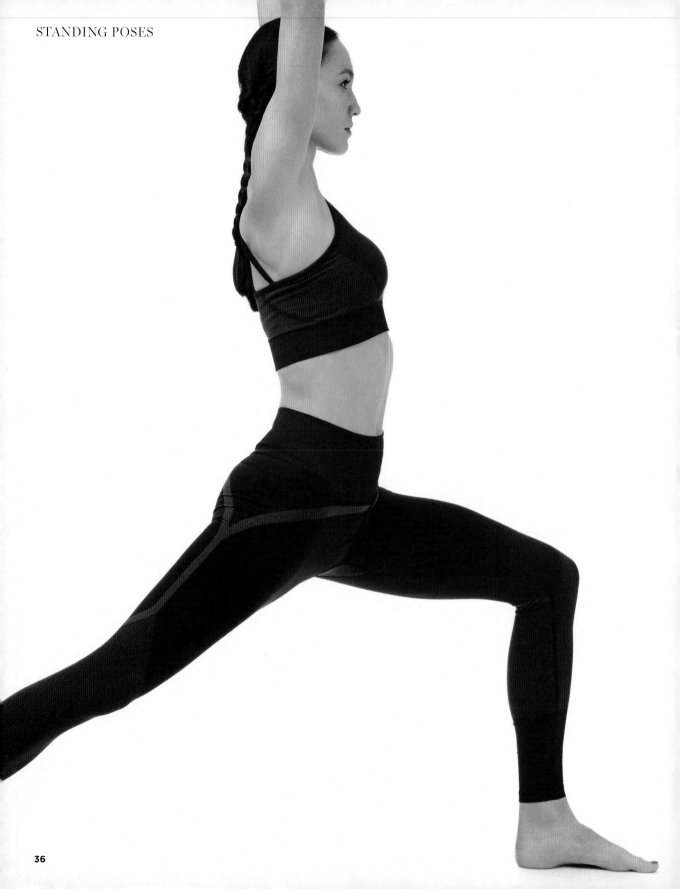

STANDING

Now that you've understood the basics, it's time to get started. We begin with *standing poses* as they form the bedrock of your asana practice. Standing postures strengthen your legs and feet, increase your focus, teach you how to *stabilise a pose* by grounding through your feet, and help you build the *endurance* you'll need for more complex asanas. Always remember to *prepare your body* by following the warm-up suggestions, even if you are familiar with the pose, as this will enable you find your fullest expression of the asana.

TRIANGLE
Trikonasana

Meaning: tri (three) kona (angle) – three angles make a triangle

Triangle is usually taught early on in your yoga journey. The key to doing the pose well is to extend your leading arm as far sideways as you can before lowering it towards the ground, and to use your back muscles to support the rotation of your torso to open your chest.

PREPARATION

✦ Cat/Cow (p30) ✦ Seated side bend (p30) ✦ Thread the needle (p31)

BENEFITS

MUSCLES/JOINTS
✦ Tones and strengthens your ankles
✦ Releases your hips and legs
✦ Lengthens your spine
✦ Opens the sides of your body

PHYSIOLOGICAL
✦ Develops your chest
✦ Stimulates your internal organs

SUBTLE/THERAPEUTIC
✦ Removes stiffness in your legs and hips
✦ Relieves backache
✦ Eases neck sprains
✦ Reduces menstrual symptoms

RISKS/PRECAUTIONS

✦ Neck, lower back, knees ✦ knee issues ✦ neck problems ✦ back pain

CONTRAINDICATIONS

✦ Slipped disc ✦ back problems ✦ low blood pressure ✦ heart conditions ✦ diarrhoea

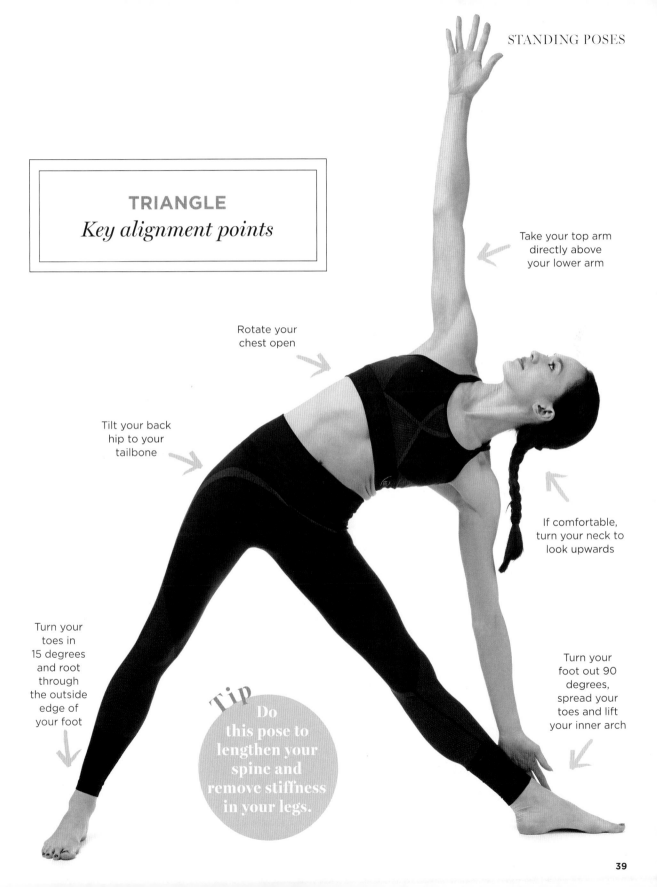

TRIANGLE
Key alignment points

Take your top arm directly above your lower arm

Rotate your chest open

Tilt your back hip to your tailbone

If comfortable, turn your neck to look upwards

Turn your toes in 15 degrees and root through the outside edge of your foot

Turn your foot out 90 degrees, spread your toes and lift your inner arch

Tip
Do this pose to lengthen your spine and remove stiffness in your legs.

Trikonasana
IN-DEPTH FORM GUIDE

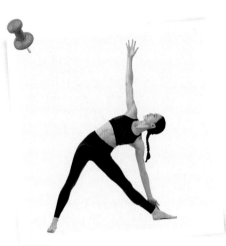

Getting into the pose

● Stand sideways on the centre of your mat and step your feet a leg's length apart.
● Turn your left foot out 90 degrees and your right foot in 15 degrees. Align your left heel to your right instep, then root down through your big and little toes, the centre of your heels and the outer edge of your right foot. Breathe.
● Place your hands on your hips and tilt your left hip down and your right hip back and up. On an inhale, extend your arms out to shoulder height, palms facing down. As you exhale, keep your arms parallel to the floor as you reach your left hand outwards as far sideways

> ❝ *Use the in-breath to ground through your feet and lengthen your side body, and out-breath to release into the twist* ❞

as is comfortable. Exhale, then breathe again, reach further forwards with your arms parallel to the floor before releasing your left hand down to rest where it naturally lands, on your calf or ankle.
● On your next inhale, float your right arm overhead and rotate open your

chest, so your right shoulder is above the left and your arms are in a straight line. Let your gaze rest on the floor, directly ahead or, if comfortable for your neck, turn your head to look up at your top hand.

Work in the pose

● Breathe into the pose, making micro-adjustments, until you feel rooted but open, using your in-breath to ground through your feet and lengthen your side body, and your out-breath to release further into the twist. Pull your abdominals towards your spine, inhale and lift your ribcage away from your waist. This will create space in your torso to help you rotate your chest more fully. Imagine lines of energy running from your centre and out through your limbs. Rest in your final position for five to 10 breaths, breathing deeply into your belly.

Coming out of the pose

● When you are ready, root through your feet and inhale up to standing, then exhale as you lower your arms and step your feet together. Pause for a moment to register the effects of the pose, then repeat on the other side.
● Rest in Savasana (p35) for a couple of minutes, then use the space opposite to jot down your experience and any areas you want to work on next time you practise this pose.

Modifications

Inflexible?
Place your feet closer together; keep your front leg bent; align your heels rather than your heel to your instep; place your front hand on your thigh or a chair.

Hypermobile?
Maintain a micro-bend in your front knee; don't over extend your lower back.

Injured?
Neck: look forwards not upwards. Knees: don't let your knees roll inwards; make sure your rear heel is extended.

GO DEEPER

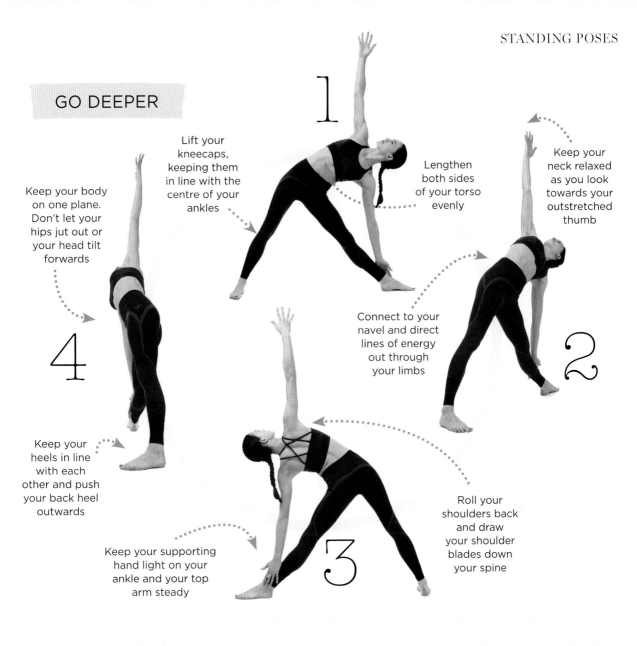

1

Lengthen both sides of your torso evenly

Keep your neck relaxed as you look towards your outstretched thumb

Lift your kneecaps, keeping them in line with the centre of your ankles

Keep your body on one plane. Don't let your hips jut out or your head tilt forwards

Connect to your navel and direct lines of energy out through your limbs

2

4

Keep your heels in line with each other and push your back heel outwards

Roll your shoulders back and draw your shoulder blades down your spine

3

Keep your supporting hand light on your ankle and your top arm steady

Practice notes   Use this space to deepen your experience of the pose, making notes on any challenges, what felt good and the areas to focus on in the future.

_____

_____

_____

_____

_____

WIDE-LEGGED STANDING FORWARD FOLD
Prasarita padottanasna

Meaning: prasarita (extended), pada (foot), ut (intense), tan (to stretch)

This pose deeply relaxes your mind and is useful to practise after challenging standing poses or balances. Keep your hamstrings safe by maintaining a micro-bend in your knees. For a more invigorating pose, interlink your fingers behind your back and raise your arms overhead as you fold forwards.

PREPARATION

✦ Cat/Cow (p30) ✦ Reclining hand to toe pose (p32) ✦ Lizard (p32)

BENEFITS

MUSCLES/JOINTS
✦ Strengthens your feet, legs and core
✦ Stretches your hamstrings and adductors (inner thighs)
✦ Lengthens your spine

PHYSIOLOGICAL
✦ Calms your brain
✦ Balances your nervous system
✦ Improves your digestion

SUBTLE/THERAPEUTIC
✦ Relieves mild backache
✦ Eases headaches
✦ Reduces fatigue
✦ Improves low blood pressure

RISKS/PRECAUTIONS
✦ Hamstrings, lower back
✦ low blood pressure ✦ lower back problems ✦ herniated disc

CONTRAINDICATIONS
✦ Detached retina ✦ glaucoma,
✦ hamstring injuries

WIDE-LEGGED STANDING FOLD
Key alignment points

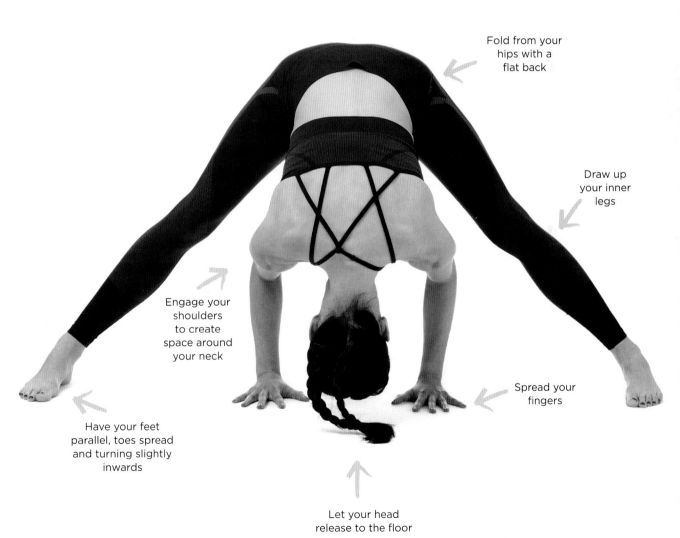

Fold from your hips with a flat back

Draw up your inner legs

Engage your shoulders to create space around your neck

Spread your fingers

Have your feet parallel, toes spread and turning slightly inwards

Let your head release to the floor

Prasarita Padottanasna
IN-DEPTH FORM GUIDE

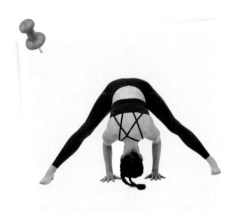

Coming into the pose

● Step your feet wide, inner edges parallel, toes spread and turned slightly inwards. Lift your inner arches by drawing your ankles away from each other, and press the outer edges of your feet and the ball of each big toe firmly into the floor.

● With your hands on your hips, inhale, root through your feet to lengthen your spine, lifting your chest, to make your front torso slightly longer than your back torso, and roll your shoulders back and down.

● As you exhale, fold forwards from your hips with a flat back, to take your spine horizontal to the floor. Place your hands directly beneath your shoulders, fingers spread. With a soft neck, continue lengthening your spine as you inhale, folding deeper as you exhale.

Work in the pose

● Draw up your kneecaps and engage your thighs, turning your inner thighs in slightly to open your sitting bones.

● Release the crown of your head towards the floor, bending your elbows but keeping your forearms vertical. Breathe deeply and evenly for five breaths,

Coming out of the pose

● Lengthen your front torso, place your hands on your hips and engage your core as you inhale to come up to standing with a flat back. Take your time to come up, especially if you suffer from dizziness or have low blood pressure.

● Notice your experience – what is challenging, what feels uplifting – then repeat the pose once or twice more, breathing consciously into any tight areas and relishing any invigorating sensations you feel. Step your feet together and pause for a moment to absorb the effects of the pose.

> ❝ *As you exhale, fold forwards from your hips with a flat back, to take your spine horizontal to the floor* ❞

Modifications

Inflexible?
Rest your forearms on your thighs or rest your hands on a wall.

Hypermobile?
Don't lock your knees; lift through your legs; engage your core.

Injured?
Back problems: place your hands on your knees, spine parallel to the floor.

GO DEEPER

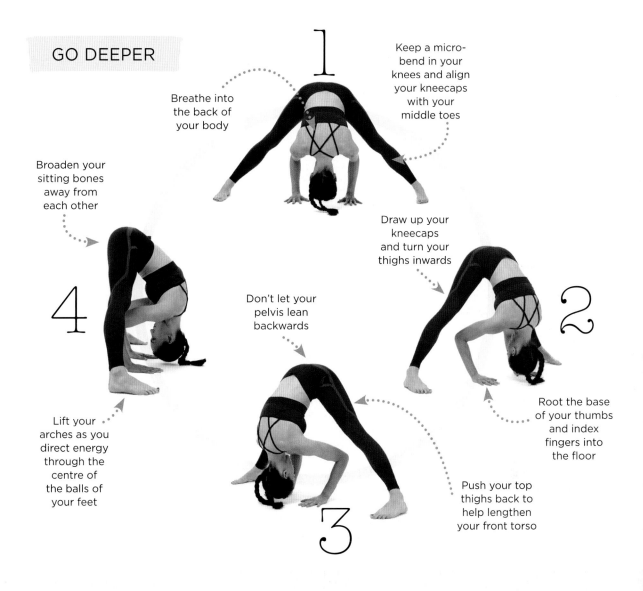

1

Keep a micro-bend in your knees and align your kneecaps with your middle toes

Breathe into the back of your body

Broaden your sitting bones away from each other

Draw up your kneecaps and turn your thighs inwards

4

Don't let your pelvis lean backwards

2

Root the base of your thumbs and index fingers into the floor

Lift your arches as you direct energy through the centre of the balls of your feet

3

Push your top thighs back to help lengthen your front torso

Practice notes   Use this space to deepen your experience of the pose, making notes on any challenges, what felt good and the areas to focus on in the future.

_____

_____

_____

_____

_____

WARRIOR I
Virabhadrasana I

Meaning: Virabhadra was a warrior created by a lock of Lord Shiva's hair which came up out of the ground

There are three Warrior poses in yoga. This first one is more intense than the more common Warrior II pose, where you face sideways onto your mat with your arms extended to shoulder height. To get the full benefits of the pose, it's important to keep you hips square to the front.

PREPARATION

✦ Puppy dog (p31) ✦ Crescent moon (p32)
✦ Reclining hand to toe (p32) (raise the leg vertically instead of to the side)

BENEFITS

MUSCLES/JOINTS
✦ Strengthens your feet, ankles, legs, upper back, shoulders and arms
✦ Opens your groin, chest and lungs
✦ Aids flexibility in your hips, back and shoulders

PHYSIOLOGICAL
✦ Develops stamina
✦ Aids deep breathing

SUBTLE/THERAPEUTIC
✦ Eases sciatica
✦ Relieves stiffness in your back, shoulders and neck
✦ Develops stability
✦ Boosts energy

RISKS/PRECAUTIONS

✦ Knees (misaligned/overextended), hips ✦ mild low/high blood pressure (do occasionally) ✦ neck (don't look up) ✦ shoulders (take arms horizontally)

CONTRAINDICATIONS

✦ High blood pressure
✦ knee problems ✦ hip issues
✦ sciatica

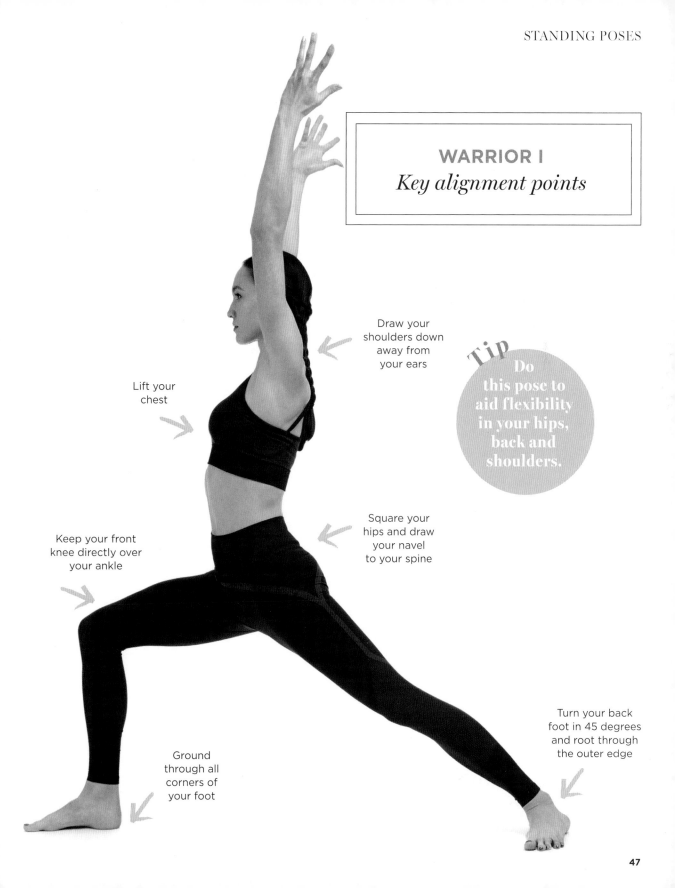

WARRIOR I
Key alignment points

Draw your shoulders down away from your ears

Tip
Do this pose to aid flexibility in your hips, back and shoulders.

Lift your chest

Keep your front knee directly over your ankle

Square your hips and draw your navel to your spine

Ground through all corners of your foot

Turn your back foot in 45 degrees and root through the outer edge

Virabhadrasana I

IN-DEPTH FORM GUIDE

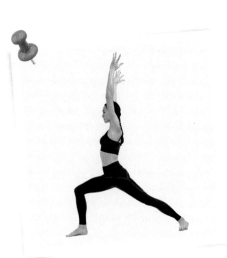

Coming into the pose
● Stand with your feet hip-width apart, inner edges parallel. Take a couple of deep breaths into your belly, allowing your weight to sink towards the earth on the out-breath. Fold forwards from your hips and place your hands either side of your feet, resting on your fingertips. Take a large step straight back with your left leg, then turn your toes out 45 degrees. Straighten your back leg and come up to standing.
● With your hands on your hips, take your left hip forwards and your right hip back to square your pelvis, then hug your

> ❝ *Take a few deep breaths into your belly, allowing your weight to sink towards the earth on the out-breath* ❞

thighs towards the centre line of your mat.
● Inhale and take your arms overhead, palms touching and thumbs interlaced. Then, as you exhale, bend your front knee until it is directly over your front ankle, aligned with your middle toes.

Ground through your big and little toes, and raise your inner arches. If it feels comfortable for your neck, take your gaze beyond your fingertips.

Work in the pose
● Keep grounding through the outside edge of your back foot and engage your front thigh muscles to lift your leg. Draw your left hip bone forwards to keep your hips square to the front of your mat. If you find it difficult to square your hips, edge your back foot slightly nearer the long side of your mat
● Bring your navel towards your spine and lengthen your torso out of your pelvis. Lift your chest as you draw your shoulder blades down your spine.
● Reach upwards through your arms at the same time as drawing your arms into your shoulder sockets.
● Breathe fully and deeply for up to 10 breaths, allowing your breath to energise the pose.

Coming out of the pose
● Inhale, and straighten your front leg. Release your arms on an exhale, step your back foot forwards and pause for a moment before repeating on the other side. When you've finished, spend a few moments in Legs up the wall (p34) to rest your legs, then when you're ready, note down your experiences of the pose in the space opposite.

Modifications

Inflexible?
Have your feet closer than a leg's distance and wider than hip-width apart; place your back heel against a wall.

Hypermobile?
Keep a micro-bend in your back knee; draw your navel towards the spine; don't sink into your hips.

Injured?
Neck: look forwards instead of upwards. Shoulders: place your hands on your hips or have your arms to your sides, upper arms parallel and forearms vertical.

GO DEEPER

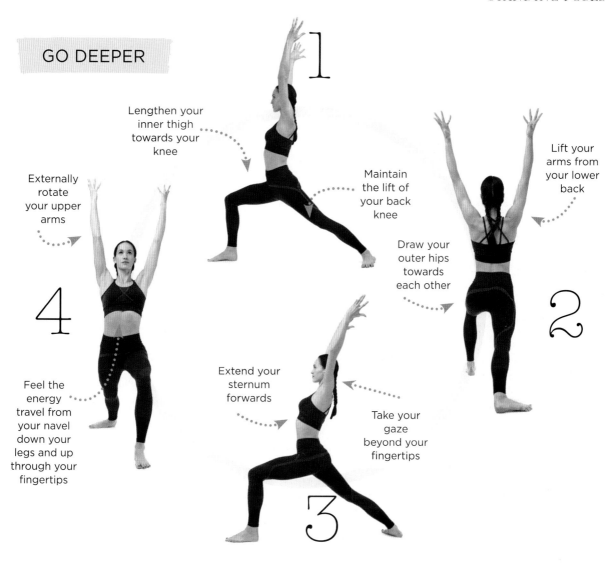

1

Lengthen your inner thigh towards your knee

Maintain the lift of your back knee

2

Lift your arms from your lower back

Draw your outer hips towards each other

3

Extend your sternum forwards

Take your gaze beyond your fingertips

4

Externally rotate your upper arms

Feel the energy travel from your navel down your legs and up through your fingertips

Practice notes

Use this space to deepen your experience of the pose, making notes on any challenges, what felt good and the areas to focus on in the future.

_____

_____

_____

_____

_____

PYRAMID
Parsvottanasana with pashima namaskarasna

Meaning: parsva (side), ut (intense), tan (to stretch), pashima (west), namaskar (salutation)

In Indian philosophy, the back of the body is considered the west. This strenuous pose gives an intense stretch to the whole body, particularly the west side. By placing your arms in reverse namaste, you open your wrists and shoulders. As a forward bend, it's also calming for your mind.

PREPARATION

✦ Cat/Cow (p30) ✦ Cow face pose (p31) ✦ Crescent moon (p32)

BENEFITS

MUSCLES/JOINTS
✦ Strong stretch for your hamstrings, glutes, back, shoulders and wrists
✦ Increases flexibility in your hips, spine and shoulders
✦ Opens your chest
✦ Strengthens your legs

PHYSIOLOGICAL
✦ Aids deep breathing
✦ Develops your balance and stamina

SUBTLE/THERAPEUTIC
✦ Calms your mind
✦ Eases respiratory complaints
✦ Relieves rounded shoulders
✦ Aids stiff legs and hips

RISKS/PRECAUTIONS

✦ Hamstrings ✦ lower back ✦ wrists and elbows ✦ low blood pressure
✦ mild high blood pressure

CONTRAINDICATIONS

✦ High blood pressure ✦ pulled hamstrings
✦ rotator cuff injury ✦ sciatica
✦ hip and spinal injuries

PYRAMID
Key alignment points

Tip
This pose stretches your hamstrings, glutes, back, shoulders and wrists.

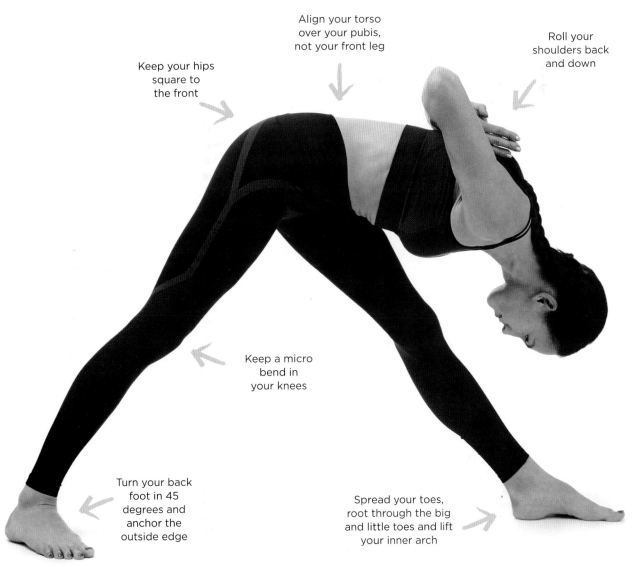

Align your torso over your pubis, not your front leg

Roll your shoulders back and down

Keep your hips square to the front

Keep a micro bend in your knees

Turn your back foot in 45 degrees and anchor the outside edge

Spread your toes, root through the big and little toes and lift your inner arch

Parsvottanasana with pashima namaskarasna
IN-DEPTH FORM GUIDE

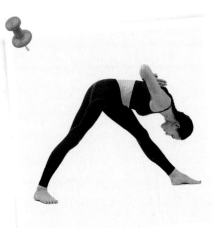

Coming into the pose

● With your feet parallel and hip-width apart, take a large step straight back with your right leg. Keeping your left foot as it is, pivot on your right heel so your foot is at a 45 degree angle. Spread your toes and root through your left big toe and the outer edge of your right foot. Lift your inner arches by drawing your ankles apart.

● With your hands on your hips, bring your right hip forwards and your left hip back, so your pelvis is facing the front of your mat. If your hips aren't quite square, take your right foot slightly nearer the long edge of your mat. Draw your inner thighs towards each other to stabilise the pose.

● Take your arms into reverse prayer, inching your hands up between your shoulder blades. Alternatively, clasp your elbows, forearms or wrists behind your back. Inhale and root down to the ground as you lengthen your spine

> *Root through your feet, firming your legs and engaging your core as you lengthen your spine through the crown*

then, on an exhale, fold forwards from your hips, keeping your spine flat. Travel slowly and mindfully until you reach the end of your out-breath, then pause.

● On your next inhale, extend and lengthen your entire spine, then gently release on an exhale to fold further forwards over your pubis, letting your back naturally curve as you get lower. Continue lengthening and lowering in this way as far as is comfortable.

Work in the pose

● Work on maintaining your sense of being grounded, rooting through your feet, firming your legs and engaging your core as you lengthen your spine through the crown of your head. Draw your shoulder blades down your back.

● Keep your sacrum level by making sure your pelvis is square, drawing your left hip back and your right hip forwards.

● This pose can feel quite meditative. Rest here for five to 10 breaths, breathing evenly through your nose, allowing your mind to soften and be still.

Coming out of the pose

● When you feel ready, root through your feet and inhale to return to standing, then exhale to step your feet together. Pause for a moment, then repeat on the other side. Take a rest in Legs up the wall (p34), then make notes on your experience.

Modifications

Inflexible?
Bend your front knee slightly; place your hands on a wall or on blocks either side of your front foot; place your back heel against a wall; take your feet wider than hip-distance apart; clasp your elbows or forearms behind your back.

Hypermobile?
Don't lock your knees; engage your core.

Injured?
Low blood pressure? Come out of the pose slowly. Mild high blood pressure? Place your hands against a wall. Hip conditions? Don't bend as low.

GO DEEPER

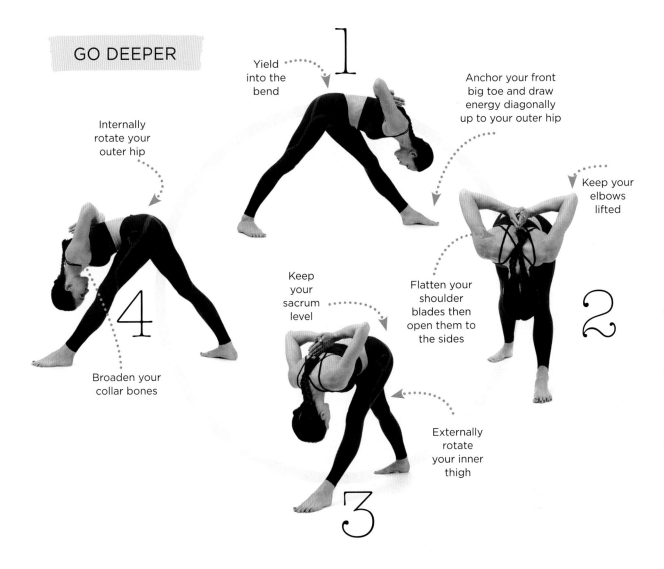

Yield into the bend

Anchor your front big toe and draw energy diagonally up to your outer hip

Keep your elbows lifted

Internally rotate your outer hip

Keep your sacrum level

Flatten your shoulder blades then open them to the sides

Broaden your collar bones

Externally rotate your inner thigh

1

2

3

4

Practice notes Use this space to deepen your experience of the pose, making notes on any challenges, what felt good and the areas to focus on in the future.

_____

_____

_____

_____

_____

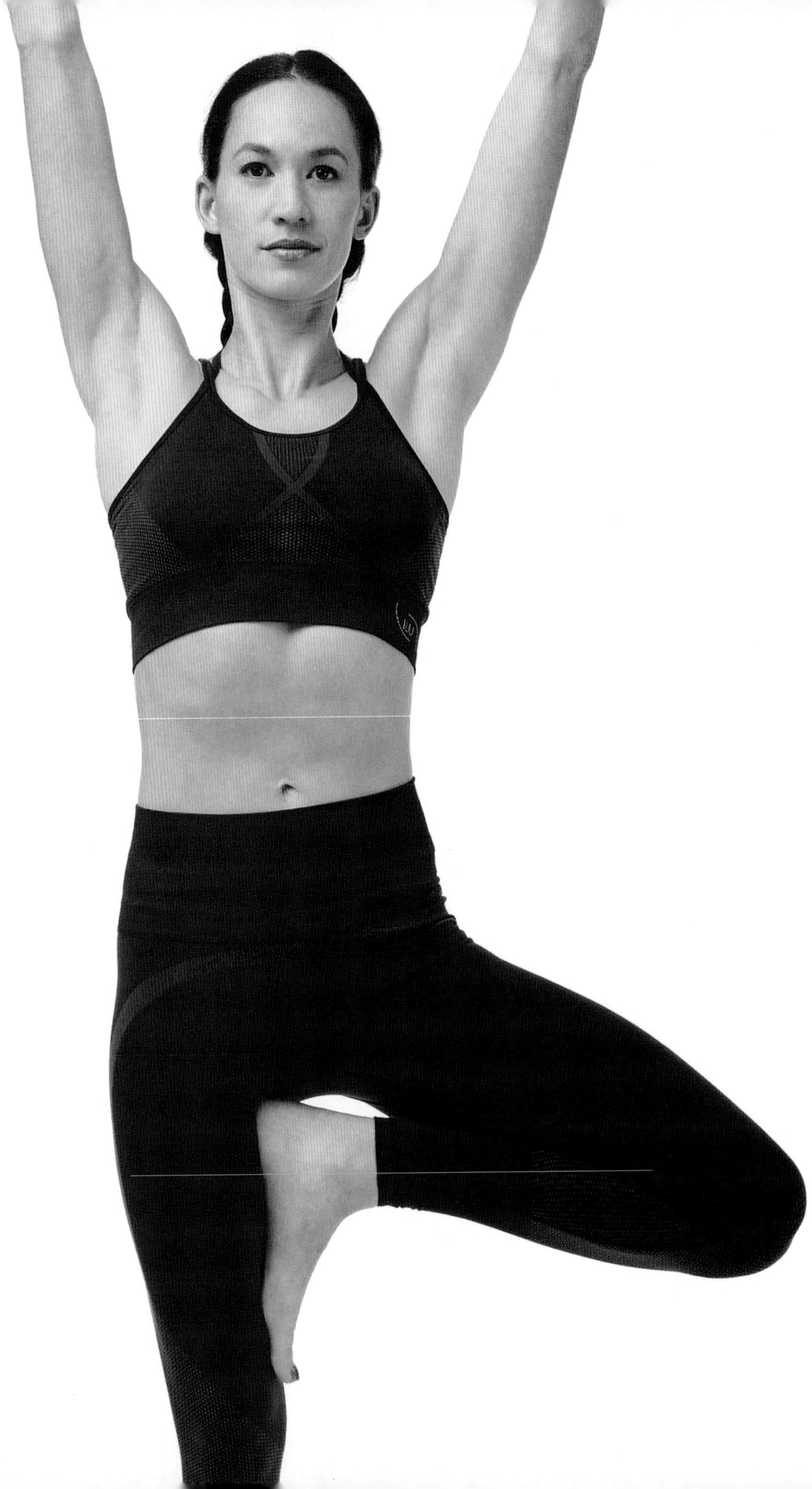

BALANCES

Having learnt how to *ground your body* through your feet in standing asanas, you'll find the balance poses in this chapter much easier. Balances bring a beautiful sense of *serenity to your practice*, and as you learn to find stillness on your mat, this is often translated into your life in general. Allow yourself to be *soft in the poses* – balance isn't about holding on rigidly but gently oscillating between two positions until you find the place of perfect equanimity. Focusing on a point in the distance will *help stabilise* you and keep your energy rooting into the earth.

TREE
Vrksasana

Meaning: vrksa (tree)

Trees sway in the wind, so in Tree pose allow your body to fluctuate gently with your breath. You'll find steadiness by rooting down through your supporting leg and pressing the sole of your foot into your inner thigh while pressing your thigh into your sole.

PREPARATION

✦ Seated side bend (p30) ✦ Lizard (p32) ✦ Boat (p33)

BENEFITS

MUSCLES/JOINTS
✦ Tones your legs and shoulder muscles
✦ Strengthens your feet, ankles, legs and core
✦ Increases the flexibility of your hips and knees
✦ Stretches groin, inner thighs

PHYSIOLOGICAL
✦ Aids physical and mental balance
✦ Develops stability

SUBTLE/THERAPEUTIC
✦ Calms your nerves
✦ Focuses your mind
✦ Aids grounding
✦ Helps cultivate patience

RISKS/PRECAUTIONS

✦ Knees ✦ low blood pressure ✦ high blood pressure (keep hands in prayer position) ✦ foot and ankle conditions

CONTRAINDICATIONS

✦ Headache ✦ serious foot and ankle conditions

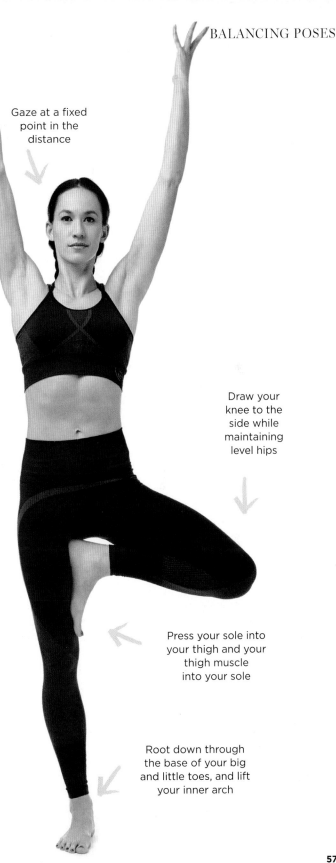

TREE
Key alignment points

Gaze at a fixed point in the distance

Extend your arms overhead, palms facing each other

Draw your knee to the side while maintaining level hips

Balance your weight centrally over your right leg and foot

Press your sole into your thigh and your thigh muscle into your sole

Root down through the base of your big and little toes, and lift your inner arch

Tip
Do this pose to develop stability and to focus your mind.

Vrksasana
IN-DEPTH FORM GUIDE

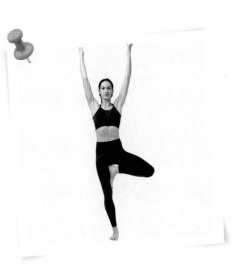

Coming into the pose

● Stand with your feet hip-distance apart and take two or three slow deep breaths to centre yourself, then transfer your weight so that it's centred over your right leg, your knee and hip stacked over your foot. Spread your toes and ground through the base of your big and little toes. Lift the inner arch of your foot.

● Keeping a micro-bend in your supporting knee, focus on a fixed point ahead and grasp your left ankle, placing the sole of your left foot against your inner right thigh or calf (avoid the knee area or you could sustain an injury). Rest your hands on your hips.

● Keeping your hips square to the front, open your left knee out to the side, and bring your hands together in prayer position at your heart.

Work in the pose

● Using ujayi breathing (p23) throughout, press the sole of your left foot into your right thigh and engage your thigh to anchor your foot. Allow your weight to release through your right leg and foot, yielding into the ground as you feel a corresponding lift upwards through your body.

● If you feel balanced here, on your next inhale, draw your shoulder blades down your back as you slowly glide your hands overhead, palms facing each other, elbows close to your ears.

● Finding a balance between steadiness and ease, breathe calmly in the pose for up to two minutes.

Coming out of the pose

● When you feel ready, exhale and, with control, gently lower your hands and foot to return to standing. Pause for a moment with your feet together before repeating on the other side. As you're only in the pose a relatively short time, repeat the balance on both sides, perhaps experimenting with closed eyes if you want a stronger challenge, then rest in Savasana (p35) before writing up your experience.

> ❝ *Finding a balance between steadiness and ease, breathe calmly in the pose for up to two minutes* ❞

Modifications

Inflexible?
Stand with your back near/against a wall; place your raised foot on your inner calf.

Hypermobile?
Engage your thighs and core; maintain a micro-bend in the supporting knee.

Injured?
Knees: rest the heel of your raised foot above your ankle, toes on the floor. Shoulders: use prayer hands. Back: rest against a wall; keep your hips in neutral.

GO DEEPER

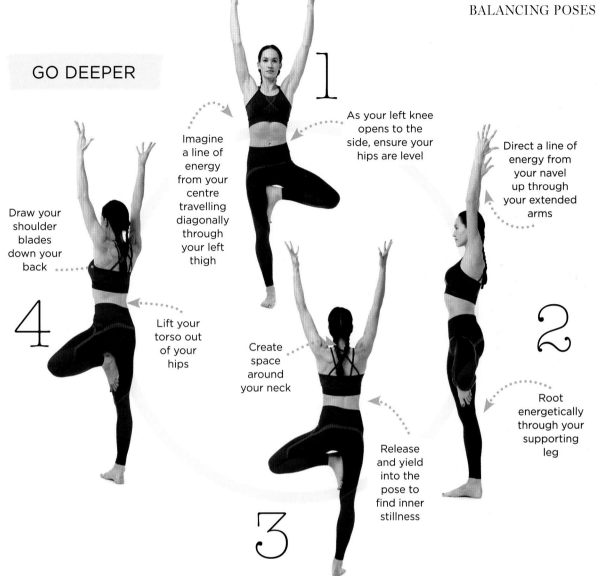

1

As your left knee opens to the side, ensure your hips are level

Imagine a line of energy from your centre travelling diagonally through your left thigh

Draw your shoulder blades down your back

4

Lift your torso out of your hips

Create space around your neck

3

Release and yield into the pose to find inner stillness

2

Direct a line of energy from your navel up through your extended arms

Root energetically through your supporting leg

Practice notes   Use this space to deepen your experience of the pose, making notes on any challenges, what felt good and the areas to focus on in the future.

_____

_____

_____

_____

_____

EAGLE
Garudasana

Meaning: Garuda (mythical king of the birds)

Eagle is a strong pose that requires and builds inner and outer strength, flexibility and endurance. It can be challenging for beginners, so if it's new to you, practise the arms and legs separately. Once you become familiar with Eagle, it can bring a wonderful sense of stillness and focus.

PREPARATION

✦ Thread the needle (p31) ✦ Cow face pose (p31) ✦ Bicycle twist (p33)

BENEFITS

MUSCLES/JOINTS	PHYSIOLOGICAL	SUBTLE/THERAPEUTIC
✦ Stretches your upper back and thighs ✦ Tones your nerves ✦ Aids flexibility of your knees, hips and shoulders ✦ Stretches your ankles and calves	✦ Improves your balance ✦ Builds stamina	✦ Eases sciatica ✦ Relieves rheumatism ✦ Aids asthma ✦ Eases lower back pain

RISKS/PRECAUTIONS

✦ Knees and shoulders ✦ mild knee and shoulder issues

CONTRAINDICATIONS

✦ Knee and shoulder injuries

EAGLE
Key alignment points

Press your palms together

Gaze at a fixed point in front of you

Cross your right elbow over your left and wrap your forearms together

Lower yourself down as if you're sitting on an imaginary chair

Wrap your right thigh over your left and hook your foot in behind your calf

Press into all four corners of your foot

Tip
This pose stretches your upper back and thighs and aids asthma.

61

Garudasana
IN-DEPTH FORM GUIDE

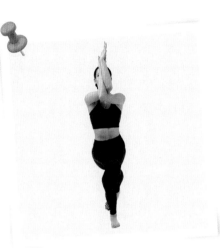

Getting into the pose

● Stand with your feet hip-distance apart and take a few moments to feel connected to the earth. Lift your toes, spread them wide, then float them back down to the ground. Root through your big and little toes, lift your arches and let the weight of your body sink into your feet. Breathe.

● When you feel grounded, take your weight onto your left foot, bend your left knee and place your right thigh over your left, then wrap your right shin behind your left calf, hooking your toes right round. Gaze on a fixed point ahead to aid your balance.

● Softly inhale as you float your arms out to the sides to shoulder height. On an exhale, cross your arms in front of you, right elbow on top of left, then intertwine your forearms to bring your palms together, thumbs facing you and fingertips pointing up.

Work in the pose

● With your forearms vertical, draw your shoulder blades down your spine, and raise your elbows to open up the space between your shoulder blades.

● Slowly and with control, begin to bend your left knee and lower your body, as if you're sitting on an imaginary chair.

● Use ujjayi breathing (p23) to help you stay focused and balanced. Notice if you can keep your mind open and relaxed, despite your body being asymmetrical and twisted. Rest in the pose for 15 to 20 seconds.

Coming out of the pose

● When you feel ready, exhale as you gently to unfurl your body. Pause with your feet together for a few moments, then repeat on the other side, practising up to three rounds on each side before resting in Legs up the wall (p34), and writing up what you have learned.

> ❝ *Notice if you can keep your mind open and relaxed, despite your body being asymmetrical and twisted* ❞

Modifications

Inflexible?
Place the backs of your hands together or extend your arms in front of you holding a strap between your hands. Cross your thighs, but place the toe of your raised foot on the floor, not behind your calf.

Hypermobile?
Actively engage your leg, arm and shoulder muscles.

Injured?
Knees: practise arms only and lower with your knees together. Shoulders: practise legs only and place your hands on your hips or in prayer.

GO DEEPER

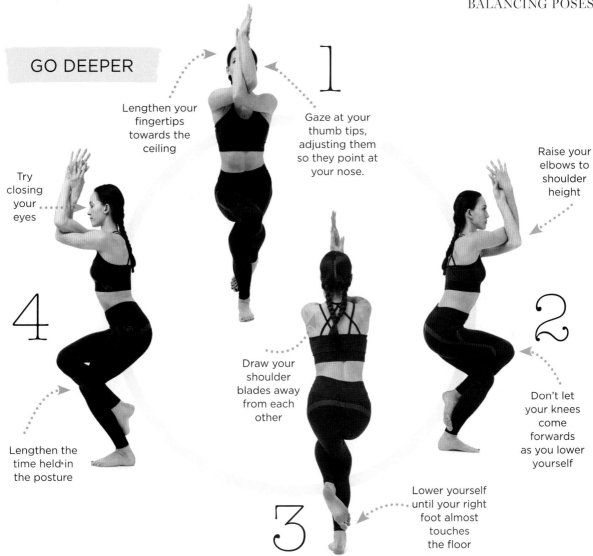

1

Gaze at your thumb tips, adjusting them so they point at your nose.

Lengthen your fingertips towards the ceiling

Raise your elbows to shoulder height

Try closing your eyes

4

Lengthen the time held in the posture

Draw your shoulder blades away from each other

2

Don't let your knees come forwards as you lower yourself

Lower yourself until your right foot almost touches the floor

3

Practice notes Use this space to deepen your experience of the pose, making notes on any challenges, what felt good and the areas to focus on in the future.

_____

_____

_____

_____

_____

HALF MOON
Ardha chandrasana

Meaning: ardha (half), chandra (moon)

This is a beautiful pose that is quietly energising. Rather than contracting your muscles to help you focus, you'll find it easier to balance if you focus on directing your energy out through your limbs. Aim to have 30-40 per cent of your weight in your front hand.

PREPARATION

✦ Reclining hand to toe (p32) ✦ Lizard (p32) ✦ Bicycle twist (p33)

BENEFITS

MUSCLES/JOINTS
✦ Opens your ribcage, chest and shoulders
✦ Tones your lower spine and nerves of your leg muscles
✦ Strengthens your knees, legs and buttocks
✦ Increases hip flexibility

PHYSIOLOGICAL
✦ Enhances breathing
✦ Increases blood flow to your liver (standing on right leg) and your spleen and stomach (standing on left leg)

SUBTLE/THERAPEUTIC
✦ Improves your balance, co-ordination and focus
✦ Eases stress and anxiety
✦ Calms digestive problems
✦ Reduces fatigue

RISKS/PRECAUTIONS

✦ Supporting leg (knee and hip) ✦ neck
✦ minor back injury and mild hip conditions
✦ low blood pressure ✦ hamstring tears

CONTRAINDICATIONS

✦ Migraine ✦ insomnia ✦ varicose veins
✦ diarrhoea ✦ herniated disc
✦ serious back or hip injury

HALF MOON
Key alignment points

Extend through to your fingertips

Stack your top hip over your lower hip

Stack your top shoulder over your lower shoulder

Flex your ankle and spread your toes

Tip
This pose tones your lower spine and increases hip flexibility.

Place your hand about a foot in front of your supporting leg and slightly to the outside

Spread your toes, ground through your big and little toes and raise your inner arch

Ardha chandrasana
IN-DEPTH FORM GUIDE

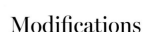

Coming into the pose

● From Triangle pose to the right (p38), step your back foot in slightly, bend your right knee and place your right fingertips about a foot in front and slightly outside of your right foot. If you have the flexibility, lower onto your palm, fingers spread and middle finger pointing forwards. Ground through the base of your index finger and thumb and lift the centre of your palm to create a kind of suction effect.

● Keeping your right leg bent, place your left hand on your left hip and root

> 66 *Experiment with balancing on your fingertips and on the palm of your hand. What difference do you notice?* 99

through your right foot as you lean into the floor until your left leg feels 'empty'. Inhale as you float your left leg up until it forms a straight line with your torso. Flex your left ankle, spread your toes and extend through the ball of the foot. Exhale.

● Inhale and root your right foot into the floor as you straighten your supporting leg and exhale to rotate your

chest and pelvis open to the left, until your hips and shoulders are stacked one above the other.

● Keeping your gaze soft towards the floor, inhale and raise your left hand up to the ceiling. Then, if comfortable for your neck, direct your gaze to your upper hand.

Work in the pose

● Breathing deeply and mindfully, feel your abdomen, front and back chest and side ribs expand as you fill out the shape you now are. Draw your shoulder blades down your back and your navel to your spine. Continue rooting through your supporting hand and foot as you feel the corresponding lift away from the floor.

● Experiment with balancing on your fingertips and on the palm of your hand. What difference do you notice? You can also temporarily wrap your top arm behind your back and nestle your fingertips around your supporting thigh to work on rotating your chest open.

● Rest in the pose as long as feels comfortable for you.

Coming out of the pose

● Exhale as you bend your right leg and lower your left leg. Pivot round into Wide-legged standing forward fold (p42) to rest for a moment before repeating on the other side. Finally, rest in Savasana (p35) for a few moments before writing up your experience.

Modifications

Inflexible?
Use a block under your supporting hand; keep your front knee bent; place your upper hand on your hip.

Hypermobile?
Don't lock your supporting knee; engage your leg muscles and core.

Injured?
Back: rest your back against a wall; don't allow it to curve. Neck: keep your neck in line with your spine or look down. Wrist: rest your lower hand (or fingertips) on a block.

GO DEEPER

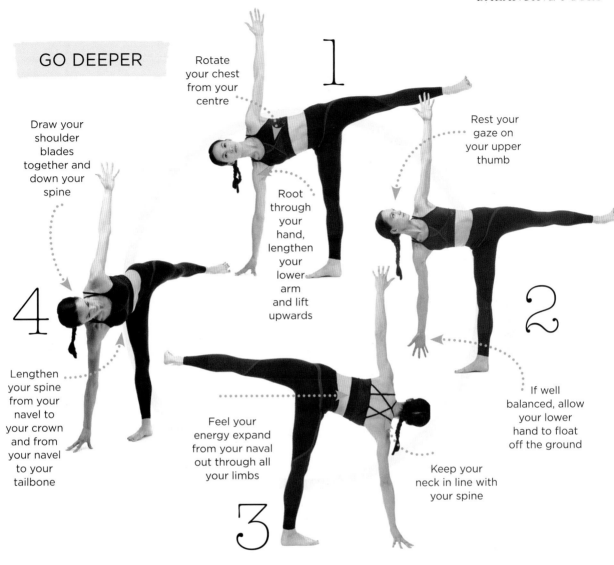

1

Rotate your chest from your centre

Rest your gaze on your upper thumb

Root through your hand, lengthen your lower arm and lift upwards

Draw your shoulder blades together and down your spine

2

If well balanced, allow your lower hand to float off the ground

4

Lengthen your spine from your navel to your crown and from your navel to your tailbone

Feel your energy expand from your naval out through all your limbs

Keep your neck in line with your spine

3

Practice notes

Use this space to deepen your experience of the pose, making notes on any challenges, what felt good and the areas to focus on in the future.

_____

_____

_____

_____

_____

LORD OF THE DANCE
Natarajasana

Meaning: nata (dancer), raja (lord or king)

Dancer can be a challenging pose, so make sure you feel comfortable in the previous balances before you try it. You'll need strong legs and good flexibility in your hips, but if you work slowly and mindfully, focusing on correct form from your feet upwards, you'll remain safe and well aligned.

PREPARATION

✦ Crescent moon (p32) ✦ Cow face pose (p31) ✦ Lizard (p32)

BENEFITS

MUSCLES/JOINTS
✦ Opens your shoulders and chest
✦ Stretches your thighs and groin
✦ Strengthens your legs and ankles
✦ Increases suppleness in your legs

PHYSIOLOGICAL
✦ Balances your nervous system

SUBTLE/THERAPEUTIC
✦ Improves your balance
✦ Aids focus
✦ Develops control of your body

RISKS/PRECAUTIONS
✦ Lower back ✦ knees
✦ hamstrings

CONTRAINDICATIONS
✦ Slipped disc
✦ carpel tunnel syndrome

LORD OF THE DANCE
Key alignment points

Grasp the outside edge of your raised foot

Focus on a point a few feet in front of you, at eye level

Keep your hips square to the front of your mat

Extend your arm in front of you and bring your thumb and index finger together

Tip

Do this pose to strengthen your legs and ankles and aid focus.

Keep your standing leg strong without locking your kneecap

Spread your toes, root through your big and little toes and raise the inner arch of your foot

Natarajasana
IN-DEPTH FORM GUIDE

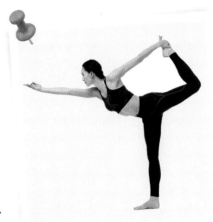

Coming into the pose

● Stand with your feet hip-distance apart and take two or three slow deep breaths to centre yourself, then transfer your weight so that it's centred over your right leg, your knee and hip stacked over your foot. Spread your toes and ground through the base of your big and little toes. Lift the inner arch of your foot.

● Keeping a micro-bend in your supporting knee, focus on a fixed point ahead and bend your left leg behind you, taking your foot to your left buttock. Grasp the outside edge of your foot with your left hand. Keeping your hips level, exhale as you slowly raise and stretch your left leg directly behind your body.

On an inhale, extend your right arm forwards to shoulder height, palm upwards, thumb and index finger forming a ring and your remaining fingers extended.

Work in the pose

● Root through your supporting foot to feel the corresponding lift throughout your whole body. Make the pose active. Press your left foot away from your left hand as you pull your hand back towards your body. Draw your left hip forwards and down to keep your pelvis level. Engage your core and lift your chest. Draw your shoulder blades down your spine as you lengthen the back of your neck.

● Feel your breath expanding your chest. Extend the energy from your centre through all your limbs. Be strong, be still. Find the balance between steadiness and ease, and rest calmly in the pose as long as you feel centred, for up to 30 seconds.

Coming out of the pose

● When you feel ready, exhale and, with control, gently lower your hands and foot to return to standing. Pause for a moment with your feet together before repeating on the other side. As you're only in the pose for a relatively short time, repeat the balance on both sides, noticing if it feels different in any way. Then rest in Savasana (p35) before writing up your experience.

> 66 *Feel your breath expanding your chest. Extend the energy from your centre through all your limbs. Be strong* 99

Modifications

Inflexible?
Warm up longer; rest your free hand against a wall or loop a strap round your raised foot and hold each end in one hand with your hands behind your neck, upper arms close to your ears and elbows pointing to the ceiling, walk your hands down the strap as flexibility increases.

Hypermobile?
Maintain a micro-bend in the supporting knee; engage your core to support your lower back; draw your arms into their sockets.

Injured?
Avoid Dancer pose.

GO DEEPER

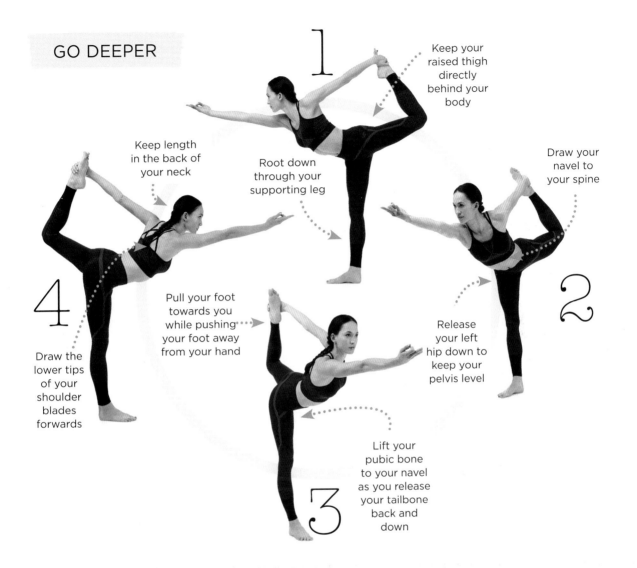

1

Keep your raised thigh directly behind your body

Keep length in the back of your neck

Root down through your supporting leg

Draw your navel to your spine

Pull your foot towards you while pushing your foot away from your hand

Release your left hip down to keep your pelvis level

2

4

Draw the lower tips of your shoulder blades forwards

Lift your pubic bone to your navel as you release your tailbone back and down

3

Practice notes

Use this space to deepen your experience of the pose, making notes on any challenges, what felt good and the areas to focus on in the future.

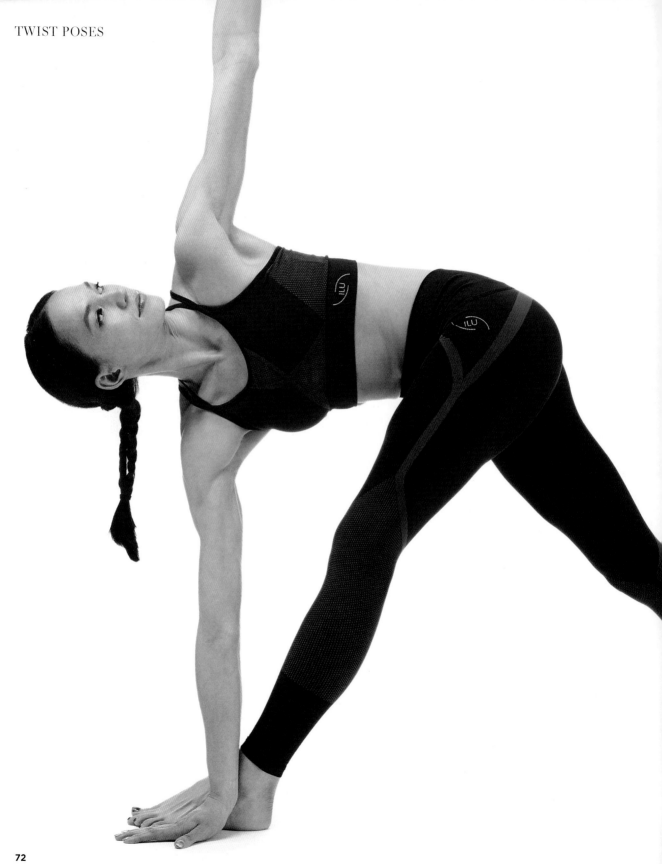

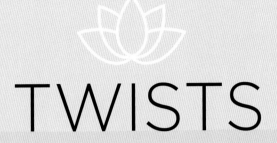

TWISTS

Twists are the ideal poses to practise when you want to *detox your system*. By compressing and then releasing the organs of your torso, you'll allow new blood to flood the area, carrying with it fresh *oxygen* and a wealth of nutrients. At the same time, waste materials from your cells rush into your *blood stream* to be carried away for processing. The key to twisting well is first to *lengthen your spine*, making more space for your individual vertebra to move, then as you exhale, release into the twist.

SAGE'S POSE I
Marichyasana I

Meaning: Marichi was a sage and the son of Brahma

There are several sage poses. This version is an open twist, where you turn your body away from your raised knee, but in others you fold your body forwards or twist it towards your raised knee. For the full benefits, focus on lengthening your spine and breathing fully into your ribcage.

PREPARATION

✦ Cat/Cow (p30) ✦ Seated side bend (p30) ✦ Thread the needle (p31)

BENEFITS

MUSCLES/JOINTS
✦ Strengthens your spine
✦ Stretches your shoulders
✦ Lengthens your spine
✦ Deep release of your back, shoulders and neck

PHYSIOLOGICAL
✦ Tones your liver, lungs and spleen
✦ Opens your chest

SUBTLE/THERAPEUTIC
✦ Stimulates your digestive organs
✦ Stimulates your brain
✦ Eases hip pain
✦ Aids detoxification

RISKS/PRECAUTIONS

✦ Lower back ✦ hamstrings ✦ bent knee ✦ neck ✦ mild back issues ✦ insomnia

CONTRAINDICATIONS

✦ High and low blood pressure ✦ sacroiliac problems ✦ disc herniation

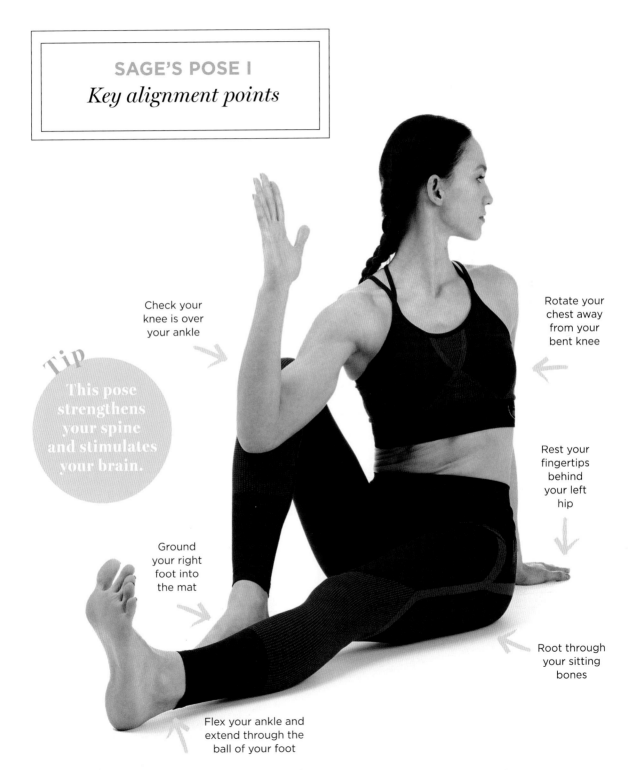

SAGE'S POSE I
Key alignment points

Tip
This pose strengthens your spine and stimulates your brain.

Check your knee is over your ankle

Rotate your chest away from your bent knee

Rest your fingertips behind your left hip

Ground your right foot into the mat

Root through your sitting bones

Flex your ankle and extend through the ball of your foot

Marichyasana I

IN-DEPTH FORM GUIDE

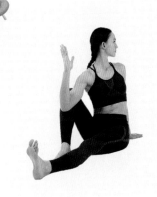

Coming into the pose

● Sit with your legs straight in front of you, feet together, ankles flexed and toes pointing to the ceiling. Rest your hands or fingertips on the floor beside your hips, fingers spread, fingertips facing forwards. Close your eyes and take a moment to become centred.

● When you feel ready, extend through the balls of your feet, spread your toes and reach through the base of your big and little toes. Lift your arches and draw the outside edges of your feet slightly towards your body. Breathe.

● Bend your right knee and place your foot a hand's distance from your left thigh, knee directly above your ankle. Root though the big and little toes of your right foot and the centre of your heel, and lift the inner arch.

● Place your left hand behind you, fingertips pointing towards the back of your mat, then inhale and raise your right arm overhead. As you exhale, lower your arm and place your outer right forearm against your inner right thigh, forearm vertical and fingers pointing to the ceiling. Inhale, and as you exhale, twist your body towards the left.

Work in the pose

● Breath softly and deeply, filling out your abdomen and ribcage, for up to one minute. As you root down through your sitting bones, feel the corresponding lift through your torso. Lengthen your spine on each inhalation, twist a little more on each exhalation, using the resistance of your forearm against your knee to help you go deeper.

● Keep your core active, by drawing your navel to your spine, and your chest open; draw your shoulders down your back. If comfortable, turn your head to gaze over your left shoulder. Breathe, and become sensitive to the sensations you are experiencing.

Coming out of the pose

● When you're ready, inhale, then exhale to return to the centre and pause for a moment before twisting momentarily to the right as a brief counter pose, then repeat on the other side.

● Rest for a few moments in Savasana (p35), then reflect on your experience of the pose, and become open to what you might like to try differently next time.

> **"**Keep the core active, by drawing your navel to your spine, and your chest open; draw your shoulders down your back**"**

Modifications

Inflexible?
Bend your left knee and tuck your foot between your buttock and right heel; wrap your right arm around the outside of the raised knee; place your rear hand against a wall.

Hypermobile?
Keep a micro-bend in your straight leg; engage your core to support your lower back.

Injured?
Disc issues: go 50 per cent into the twist, wait 24 hours. If you're fine, deepen the twist 10 per cent at a time. Insomnia: avoid after 6pm.

GO DEEPER

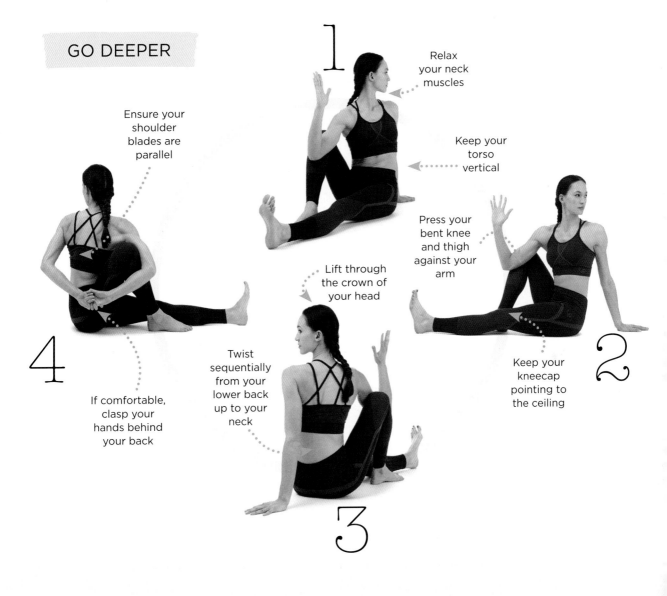

1

Relax your neck muscles

Keep your torso vertical

Press your bent knee and thigh against your arm

2

Keep your kneecap pointing to the ceiling

Ensure your shoulder blades are parallel

4

If comfortable, clasp your hands behind your back

Lift through the crown of your head

Twist sequentially from your lower back up to your neck

3

Practice notes

Use this space to deepen your experience of the pose, making notes on any challenges, what felt good and the areas to focus on in the future.

RECLINING TWIST
Supta parivartanasana II

Meaning: supta (reclining or supine), parivarta (turning or twist)

A simple twist, this pose relaxes your spine, opens your side body and massages your internal organs. To get the most out of this calming and rejuvenating pose, focus on keeping both shoulders firmly rooted into the mat rather than taking your knee to the ground.

PREPARATION

✦ Cat/Cow (p30) ✦ Seated side bend (p30) ✦ Seated twist (p30)

BENEFITS

MUSCLES/JOINTS
✦ Releases tension in your spine
✦ Opens your chest
✦ Eases stiffness in your lower back
✦ Stretches your shoulders

PHYSIOLOGICAL
✦ Hydrates your spinal discs
✦ Detoxes your digestive organs

SUBTLE/THERAPEUTIC
✦ Reduces stress
✦ Eases fatigue
✦ Helps anxiety

RISKS/PRECAUTIONS

✦ Neck issues
✦ lower back pain

CONTRAINDICATIONS

✦ Sacroiliac problems ✦ hernia
✦ disc issues

RECLINING TWIST
Key alignment points

If comfortable, turn your neck to the left

Use your hand to ease deeper into the twist

Release your bent knee over to the right

Keep your right leg active

Keep your shoulder rooting into the ground

Tip

Do this pose to ease stiffness in your lower back and reduce stress.

Flex your ankle and reach through the ball of your foot

Supta parivartanasana II

IN-DEPTH FORM GUIDE

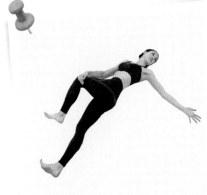

Coming into the pose

● Lie on your back, gently close your eyes and take a few moments to centre yourself, allowing your breath to deepen and your heartbeat to become slower. When you feel ready, move into the pose.

● To begin, lift your buttocks and shift them slightly to the left. This will help you maintain a healthy alignment of your spine when you're in the twist.

● Hug your knees to your chest, using your forearms to bring them close. Draw your shoulder blades down your back, and take a few breaths into your belly. After a few moments, extend your right leg to the floor, allowing your right thigh to release down to the mat.

● Rest your right hand on your bent left knee and on an exhale, gently guide it over to the right. Extend your left arm to the side, palm facing upwards and, if comfortable, gently turn your head to look to the left.

> ❝ *In your mind's eye, trace a diagonal line from your left knee to your left shoulder and lengthen your spine* ❞

Work in the pose

● Take a few moments to allow your body to acclimatise to the stretch then, breathing deeply into your left side, make any adjustments you need so that your left hip is stacked directly on top of your right. In your mind's eye, trace a diagonal line from your left knee to your left shoulder and lengthen your spine.

● Broaden your shoulder blades, expand your collar bones and create space around your neck. Breathe, and allow gravity to help you release deeper into the twist.

● Enjoy the stretch for as long as feels right for your body today, then slowly inhale back to the centre and repeat on the other side.

Coming out of the pose

● Slowly inhale back to centre and repeat on the other side, then bring your knees to your chest, take a couple of breaths and rest in Savasana (p35) for a few minutes before making any practice notes you wish to record.

Modifications

Inflexible?
If your shoulder raises off the mat, place a folded blanket or block beneath it.

Hypermobile?
Micro-bend your extended arm and leg; engage your core; don't twist to your full capacity.

Injured?
Knee: place a block or bolster beneath your bent knee. Shoulder: rest the shoulder of your extended arm on a folded blanket. Neck: don't turn your neck to the side.

GO DEEPER

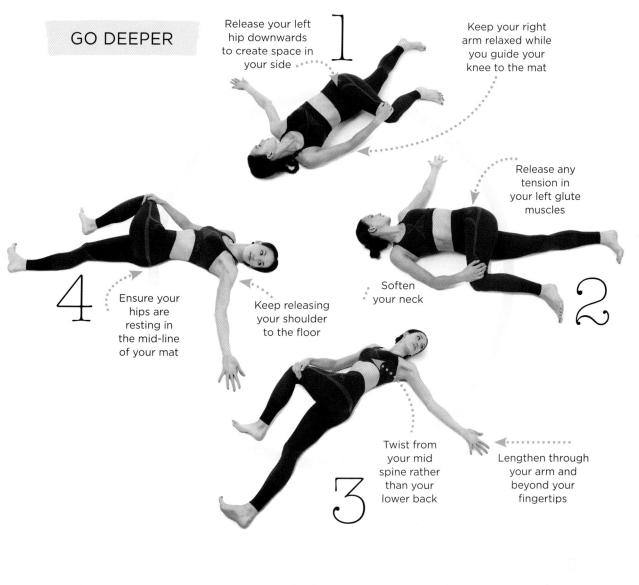

1 Release your left hip downwards to create space in your side

Keep your right arm relaxed while you guide your knee to the mat

Release any tension in your left glute muscles

Soften your neck

2

4 Ensure your hips are resting in the mid-line of your mat

Keep releasing your shoulder to the floor

Twist from your mid spine rather than your lower back

Lengthen through your arm and beyond your fingertips

3

Practice notes

Use this space to deepen your experience of the pose, making notes on any challenges, what felt good and the areas to focus on in the future.

_____

_____

_____

_____

_____

PRAYER TWIST
Parivrtta alasana

Meaning: parivrtta (revolved), alasana (high lunge)

This is a beautiful twist that focuses your mind as well as strengthens your body. It's fairly challenging and also works on your balance. It's best to practise it after you've built up the strength in your legs with the standing poses in this book, especially Warrior I (p46).

PREPARATION

✦ Cat/Cow (p30) ✦ Seated side bend (p30) ✦ Thread the needle (p31)

BENEFITS

MUSCLES/JOINTS
✦ Strengthens your legs
✦ Releases tension in your hips
✦ Increases spinal mobility
✦ Tones your core

PHYSIOLOGICAL
✦ Boosts the circulation to your abdomen
✦ Hydrates your spinal discs

SUBTLE/THERAPEUTIC
✦ Aids your balance
✦ Improves your digestion
✦ Detoxifying

RISKS/PRECAUTIONS

✦ Low backache
✦ neck or knee pain

CONTRAINDICATIONS

✦ Lower back injury ✦ disc issues
✦ serious knee injuries

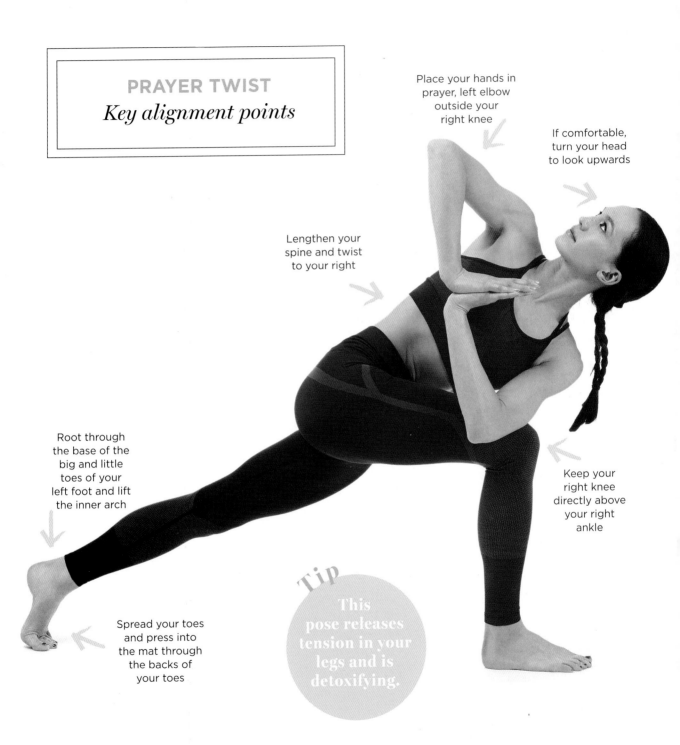

PRAYER TWIST
Key alignment points

Place your hands in prayer, left elbow outside your right knee

If comfortable, turn your head to look upwards

Lengthen your spine and twist to your right

Root through the base of the big and little toes of your left foot and lift the inner arch

Keep your right knee directly above your right ankle

Spread your toes and press into the mat through the backs of your toes

Tip

This pose releases tension in your legs and is detoxifying.

Parivrtta alasana
IN-DEPTH FORM GUIDE

Coming into the pose
● Standing with your feet hip-width apart, fold forwards from your hips and place your hands either side of your feet, resting on your fingertips. Take a large step straight back with your left leg to rest on the backs of your toes. Straighten your leg and extend through your back heel.
● Draw your navel to your spine and bring your torso up to vertical, then place your hands on your hips and take your left hip back and your right hip forwards to square your pelvis.

> " *If comfortable for your neck, turn your head to look over your right shoulder and gaze up to the ceiling* "

● With your core still engaged, inhale as you lengthen your spine out of your pelvis and draw your shoulder blades down your spine on an exhale. Inhale as you sweep your arms out to the sides and overhead and lower your hands into prayer position in front of your heart on an exhale. Then twist to the right, placing your left elbow outside your right knee.

Work in the pose
● Check that your right knee is directly over your right ankle, aligned with your middle toes. Ground through the big and little toes of your right foot and raise the inner arch. Keep extending through your back leg, lifting your thigh and reaching through to your back heel. Bring your thighs towards the mid-line.
● Rooting though your legs and drawing your right hip back, lengthen your spine on an inhale, then twist a little deeper on the exhale until you reach a soft edge. That's the point where you begin to feel resistance. Breathe into the area for a few moments and notice how it releases. When you feel ready, inhale and lengthen, then exhale and release a little further into the twist.
● If comfortable for your neck, turn your head to look over your right shoulder and gaze up to the ceiling. Breathe evenly into your belly for 30 seconds to one minute, savouring the stretch.

Coming out of the pose
● On an exhale, engage your core to come up to standing, release your arms and step your back foot forwards. Pause for a moment before repeating on the other side, then rest in Legs up the wall (p34) before writing up your experiences.

Modifications

Inflexible?
Rest both hands on your knee or put your left hand on the floor inside your right foot and right hand on your right hip until you build flexibility. Rest your back knee on the floor.

Hypermobile?
Micro-bend your back knee; firm the quads in your back leg; engage the core to protect your lower back.

Injured?
Neck pain: look ahead or down. Low back pain: don't twist deeply; place your hand on the floor (as above), or use prayer hands – don't hook your elbow outside your knee.

GO DEEPER

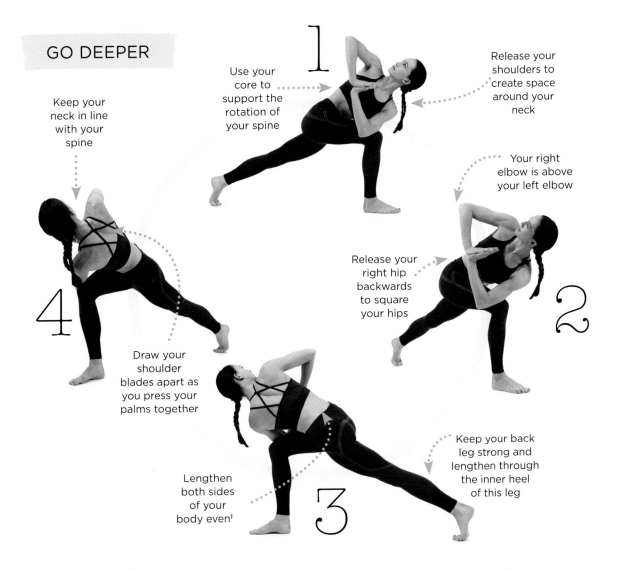

1

Use your core to support the rotation of your spine

Release your shoulders to create space around your neck

Your right elbow is above your left elbow

2

Release your right hip backwards to square your hips

Keep your neck in line with your spine

4

Draw your shoulder blades apart as you press your palms together

3

Lengthen both sides of your body even¹

Keep your back leg strong and lengthen through the inner heel of this leg

Practice notes   Use this space to deepen your experience of the pose, making notes on any challenges, what felt good and the areas to focus on in the future.

_____

_____

_____

_____

_____

REVOLVED TRIANGLE
Parivrtta trikonasana

Meaning: parivrtta (to turn around, revolve), tri (three), kona (angle)

Revolved triangle is challenging and complex, particularly for beginners. It combines a forward bend with a strong, closed twist. If it's new to you, or challenges your flexibility, focus on keeping your hips square and coming into a well aligned forward bend before working on the twist element.

PREPARATION

✦ Seated side bend (p30) ✦ Thread the needle (p31) ✦ Bicycle twist (p33)

BENEFITS

MUSCLES/JOINTS
✦ Stretches your hamstrings and glutes
✦ Opens your chest
✦ Balances your hips
✦ Increases your hip and spinal flexibility

PHYSIOLOGICAL
✦ Stimulates your abdominal organs
✦ Enhances your respiration

SUBTLE/THERAPEUTIC
✦ Aids asthma
✦ Eases low back pain
✦ Helps sciatica
✦ Improves your digestion

RISKS/PRECAUTIONS

✦ Hamstrings ✦ lower back ✦ neck
✦ headache ✦ tight hamstrings

CONTRAINDICATIONS

✦ Migraine ✦ very low blood pressure
✦ insomnia ✦ chronic back pain

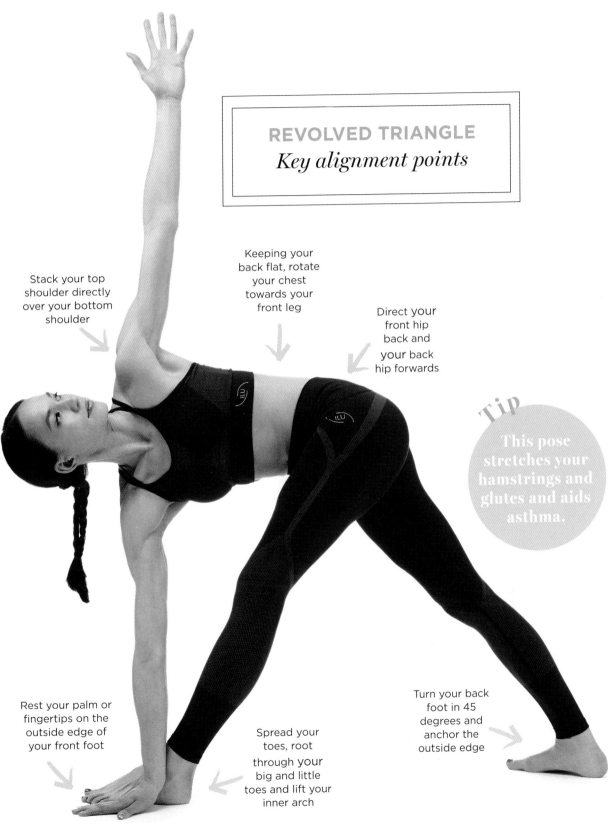

REVOLVED TRIANGLE
Key alignment points

Stack your top shoulder directly over your bottom shoulder

Keeping your back flat, rotate your chest towards your front leg

Direct your front hip back and your back hip forwards

Tip

This pose stretches your hamstrings and glutes and aids asthma.

Rest your palm or fingertips on the outside edge of your front foot

Spread your toes, root through your big and little toes and lift your inner arch

Turn your back foot in 45 degrees and anchor the outside edge

Parivrtta trikonasana
IN-DEPTH FORM GUIDE

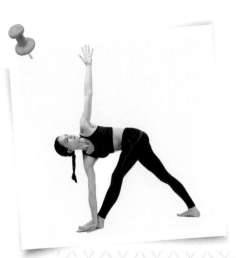

Coming into the pose
● Step your feet a little less than a leg's length apart then turn your left foot out 90 degrees and your right for in 45-60 degrees. Ground through the four corners of your front foot and lift your inner arch, and root through the outside edge of your back foot.
● Turn to face the left and square your hips so that they're parallel with the short end of your mat. Place your left hand on your left hip and, on your next inhale, raise your fight arm overhead. Keeping your hips square and rooting through both feet, as you exhale, fold forwards fromyour hips with a flat back

to take your torso parallel to the floor. Inhale, to lengthen your spine, then on exhaling, twist to the left as you release your right little finger to rest on the outside edge of your front ankle.
● Continue rotating your spine as you raise your left hand overhead, looking up at your top hand if comfortable for your neck. Breathe.

Work in the pose
● Once your body becomes acclimatised to the twist, draw your navel to your spine, and on each inhale, lengthen your torso by drawing your ribs away from your hips. On each exhale, release deeper into the twist, taking your top shoulder over your bottom shoulder.
● Use ujjayi breathing (p23) to support you in the pose, staying there for as long as feels right for you, but not for more than one minute.

Coming out of the pose
● When you feel ready, exhale, press into your back foot, release the twist and bring your torso back to upright with an inhalation. Pause for a few moments, then repeat for the same length of time with your legs reversed, twisting in the opposite direction. Afterwards, rest in Legs up the wall (p34), then make any notes you feel may be helpful for you when you next practise the pose.

> **❝** *On each exhale, release deeper into the twist, taking your top shoulder over your bottom shoulder* **❞**

Modifications
Inflexible?
Place your feet close together; keep your head in neutral or look at the floor; rest your right hand on a block; if your back rounds, rest your right hand on the inside of your front foot; practise with your back foot, right hip and right shoulder against a wall.

Hypermobile?
Maintain a micro-bend in your knees. Keep your legs, core and arms actively engaged.

Injured?
Hamstrings: bend your knees slightly. Shoulders: rest your lower arm on a brick and top hand on your upper hip. Low back pain: don't twist deeply; place your hand on the floor as above.

GO DEEPER

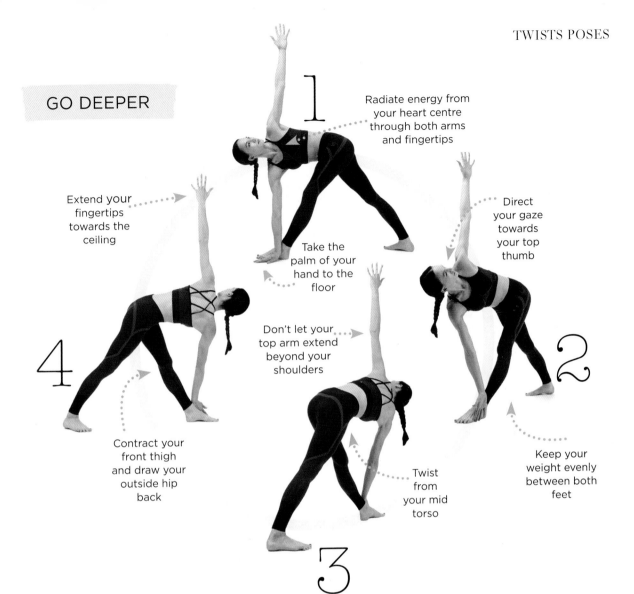

1 Radiate energy from your heart centre through both arms and fingertips

Direct your gaze towards your top thumb

Take the palm of your hand to the floor

Extend your fingertips towards the ceiling

Don't let your top arm extend beyond your shoulders

2 Keep your weight evenly between both feet

4 Contract your front thigh and draw your outside hip back

Twist from your mid torso

3

Practice notes   Use this space to deepen your experience of the pose, making notes on any challenges, what felt good and the areas to focus on in the future.

_____

_____

_____

_____

_____

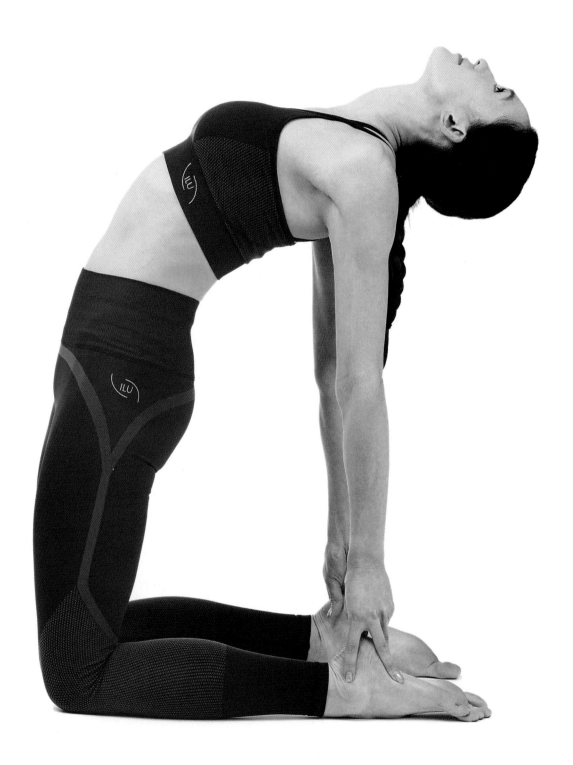

BACKBENDS

Heart-opening backbends are wonderfully invigorating, so are good to practise when you need a *boost of energy*. As with twists, think of *elongating* your spine before bending backwards and always aim to create an even curve in your spine. We've suggested you practise *shoulder* and *hip flexor stretches* before you begin, as a tight groin is likely to result in you bending from your lower back – a vulnerable area in yoga. *Engaging your core* will also help you stay safe.

ONE-LEGGED BRIDGE
Eka pada setu bandha sarvangasana

Meaning: eka(one), pada (foot), setu (bridge), bandha (lock),
sarva (all), anga (limb)

Bridge pose, where both feet remain on the ground, is often used
at the end of a practice to rebalance your body. One-legged bridge
is a challenging variation that works your core while improving your
balance and focus. It's invigorating for both your mind and your body.

PREPARATION

✦ Cat/Cow (p30) ✦ Thread the needle (p31) ✦ Crescent moon (p32)

BENEFITS

MUSCLES/JOINTS
✦ Stretches the front
of your body
✦ Strengthens your legs
and core
✦ Stabilises your hips
✦ Opens your shoulders

PHYSIOLOGICAL
✦ Calms your brain
✦ Boosts your nervous
system

SUBTLE/THERAPEUTIC
✦ Eases headaches and
period pain
✦ Aids insomnia
✦ Good for osteoporosis
✦ Helps sacroiliac problems

RISKS/PRECAUTIONS

✦ Slight neck/back pain ✦ menstruation
(stay in the pose for one minute maximum)

CONTRAINDICATIONS

✦ Hernia ✦ duodenal ulcer ✦ whiplash
✦ extreme/recent back injury

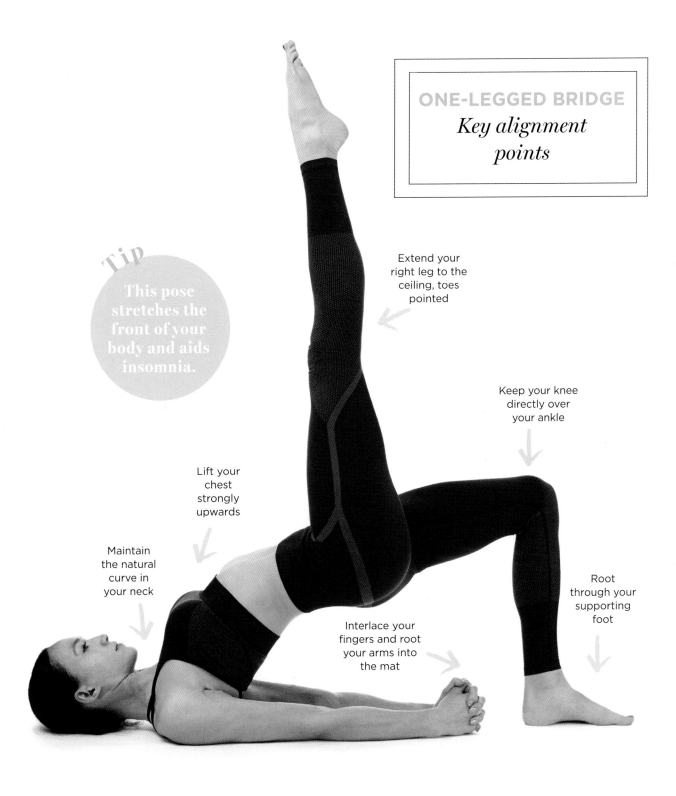

ONE-LEGGED BRIDGE
Key alignment points

Tip

This pose stretches the front of your body and aids insomnia.

Extend your right leg to the ceiling, toes pointed

Keep your knee directly over your ankle

Lift your chest strongly upwards

Maintain the natural curve in your neck

Interlace your fingers and root your arms into the mat

Root through your supporting foot

Eka pada setu bandha sarvangasana

IN-DEPTH FORM GUIDE

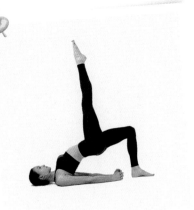

Getting into the pose

● Lie on your back with your legs straight, feet hip-distance apart, and your arms outstretched, about a foot away from your sides, palms facing upwards. Take a few moments to breathe deeply into your lower abdomen, and allow any tension in your body to softly melt away.

● When you feel ready, gently exhale and place the soles of your feet on the floor, directly beneath your knees, hip-distance apart and parallel. Check that your knees are also hip-distance apart.

> *"Press your arms into the mat, and focus on grounding through your left foot to lift through your heart"*

● Take a breath in then, on an exhale, tilt your tailbone upwards as you lift your buttocks off the floor, slowly peeling your spine away from the mat, vertebra by vertebra. Interlace your fingers and rest your hands on the floor beneath your torso, arms extended. Snuggle your shoulders together and breathe into your chest.

● On the next inhale, draw your navel to your spine and lift your right leg, foot directly over your right hip, toes pointing to the ceiling.

Work in the pose

● Roll your shoulders up, back and down, then lengthen the back of your neck. Press your arms into the mat, and focus on grounding through your left foot to lift through your heart, making sure your hips remain level.

● Draw your right leg back into your right hip socket and simultaneously extend through your right foot. Take five more deep breaths into your abdomen, filling out the shape you now are.

Coming out of the pose

● When you feel ready, on an exhale, gently and with control, lower your right leg, unclasp your fingers and take your arms to your sides. On your next exhale, slowly uncurl your spine, vertebra by vertebra, to release your spine back to the floor. Gently release your legs and place them straight on the floor, feet a comfortable distance apart.

● Rest for a moment before repeating on the other side, noticing any differences you experience on this side of your body. Spend a few moments in Savasana (p35), then make any notes you feel may help you next time you practise this pose.

Modifications

Inflexible?
Keep both legs on the floor; place your hands on your waist; rest a block beneath your sacrum.

Hypermobile?
Make sure your supporting limbs are strong – root into the ground with your foot, hands and arms; place a block between your thighs to focus on engaging them.

Injured?
Sacroiliac issues: use a block beneath your sacrum. Neck: don't lift your hips too high; start with both feet on the ground.

GO DEEPER

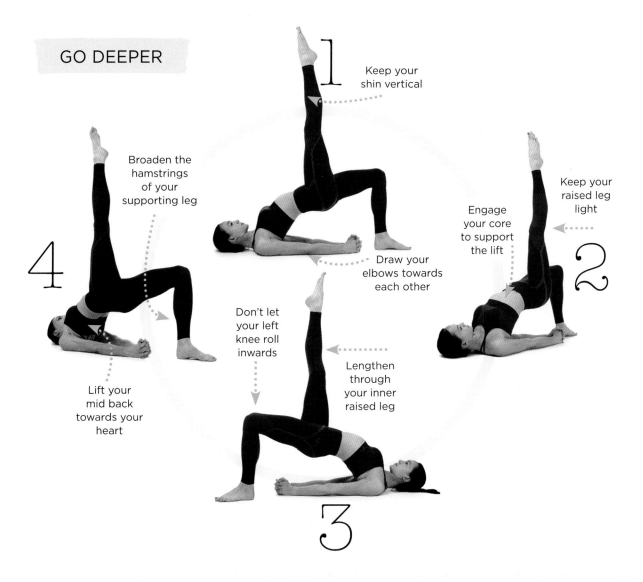

1 Keep your shin vertical

Broaden the hamstrings of your supporting leg

Keep your raised leg light

Engage your core to support the lift

4

Draw your elbows towards each other

2

Don't let your left knee roll inwards

Lengthen through your inner raised leg

Lift your mid back towards your heart

3

Practice notes

Use this space to deepen your experience of the pose, making notes on any challenges, what felt good and the areas to focus on in the future.

_____

_____

_____

_____

_____

COBRA
Bhujangasana

Meaning: bhujanga (snake or serpent)

There are three hand placements for Cobra – your hands at your lower ribs, your fingertips at the top of your shoulders or your hands further forwards and wider apart. Experiment with each (the first is the hardest), notice how your body responds and choose the one that feels right.

PREPARATION

✦ Cat/Cow (p30) ✦ Seated twist (p30) ✦ Seated side bend (p30)

BENEFITS

MUSCLES/JOINTS

✦ Strengthens your back and buttocks
✦ Tones your abdominals
✦ Strong chest opener
✦ Eases tension in your back, neck and shoulders

PHYSIOLOGICAL

✦ Tones your nervous system
✦ Increases body heat

SUBTLE/THERAPEUTIC

✦ Eases sciatica
✦ Aids hypothyroid issues
✦ Improves asthma
✦ Reduces stress

RISKS/PRECAUTIONS

✦ Mild back or wrist injuries
✦ carpel tunnel syndrome

CONTRAINDICATIONS

✦ Peptic ulcer ✦ hyperthyroidism
✦ severe back pain

COBRA
Key alignment points

Gaze forwards
with your head
aligned with
your spine

Tip
**Do
this pose
to tone your
abdominals
and open
your chest.**

Release your
shoulder blades
down your
back and
in towards
your spine

Keep your
legs active

Place your feet
hip-distance apart,
resting on the tops
of your toes

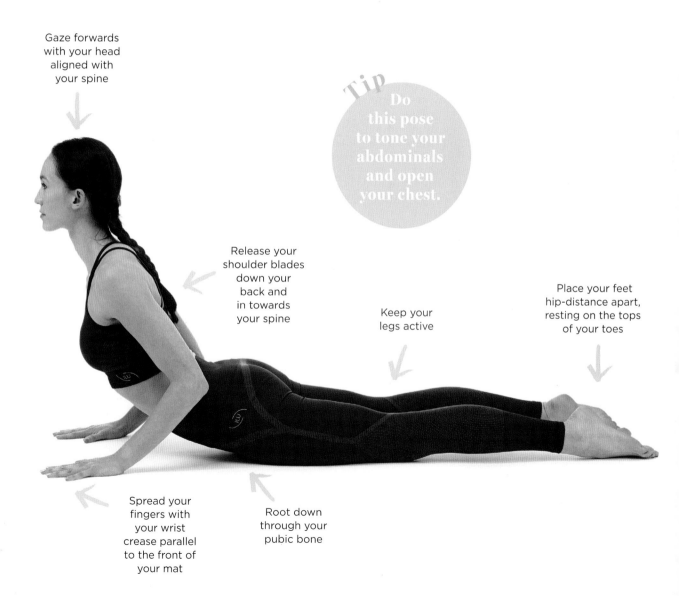

Spread your
fingers with
your wrist
crease parallel
to the front of
your mat

Root down
through your
pubic bone

Bhujangasana
IN-DEPTH FORM GUIDE

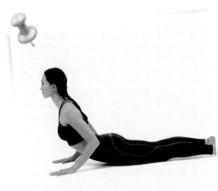

Getting into the pose

● Lie on your stomach with your forehead resting on the floor. Take a couple of deep breaths, then spread your feet hip-distance apart, ankles straight and toes spread. Straighten your legs, aligning your knees with your middle toes, and engage your inner leg muscles. Root through your pubic bone.

● Place your hands at the side of your ribs or beneath your shoulders, palms facing down, fingers spread and wrist crease parallel with the front edge of your mat.

> **" Engage your abdomen and keep rooting through your pelvic bone to extend your sacrum to your tailbone "**

● Draw your elbows together and rotate your shoulders up, back and down to create space at the base of your neck, then release your shoulder blades down your back and in towards your spine.

● Inhale, and raise your head and shoulders as far as is comfortable by drawing the back of your neck upwards, so your eyes remain looking down. Don't use your arms to assist you at this point. Exhale. On your next inhale, ground through your hands, as if you were pulling the floor towards you, and feel your chest open as you curl your spine further forwards and up, gently raising your head to take your gaze straight ahead.

Work in the pose

● Breathe into your belly and feel the shape your body is now in. Engage your abdomen and keep rooting through your pelvic bone to extend your sacrum to your tailbone. Lengthen your spine evenly without compressing your lumbar spine or the back of your neck, and see if you can feel a sense of lightness as you lift your back body.

● Breathe normally in the pose as long as feels comfortable, up to two minutes, but come out before you begin to feel any strain.

Coming out of the pose

● Slowly and with control, exhale as you lower your body to the floor one vertebra at a time and rest your head lightly on one side. If you only spent a relatively short time in the pose, say five or 10 breaths, repeat once or twice more, alternating which side of your face you rest your head. Afterwards, spend a few minutes in Savasana (p.35) to absorb the experience before making any notes you feel might be helpful.

Modifications

Inflexible?
Take your hands wider apart; turn your wrists outwards; keep the lift low initially.

Hypermobile?
Spend a shorter time in the pose; engage your core; focus on creating an even curve throughout your spine.

Injured?
Wrists: place your hands on a folded blanket; rest on your forearms; don't lift your chest too high. Low back pain: place a blanket beneath your abdomen.

GO DEEPER

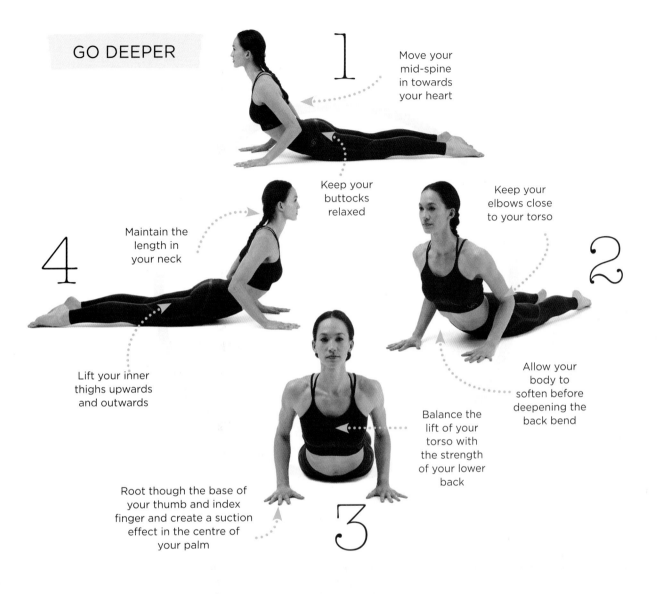

1

Move your mid-spine in towards your heart

Keep your buttocks relaxed

Keep your elbows close to your torso

4

Maintain the length in your neck

2

Lift your inner thighs upwards and outwards

Allow your body to soften before deepening the back bend

Balance the lift of your torso with the strength of your lower back

Root though the base of your thumb and index finger and create a suction effect in the centre of your palm

3

Practice notes Use this space to deepen your experience of the pose, making notes on any challenges, what felt good and the areas to focus on in the future.

_____

_____

_____

_____

_____

CAMEL
Ustrasana

Meaning: **ustra** (camel)

This uplifting pose is great to do after you've been working at a computer. By opening the front of your body and broadening your shoulders, it counteracts a hunched spine and floods your body with energy. Try it at the end of a long day or when you need a mental boost.

PREPARATION

✦ Cat/Cow (p30) ✦ Cow face pose (p31) ✦ Crescent moon (p32)

BENEFITS

MUSCLES/JOINTS

✦ Tones your back
✦ Opens your shoulders
✦ Expands your chest
✦ Increases flexibility in your spine

PHYSIOLOGICAL

✦ Boosts your lung capacity
✦ Enhances the blood flow to your organs

SUBTLE/THERAPEUTIC

✦ Regulates menstrual flow
✦ Eases abdominal cramps
✦ Improves your posture

RISK/PRECAUTIONS

✦ Neck issues

CONTRAINDICATIONS

✦ Severe constipation ✦ diarrhoea ✦ headache, migraine or high blood pressure

100

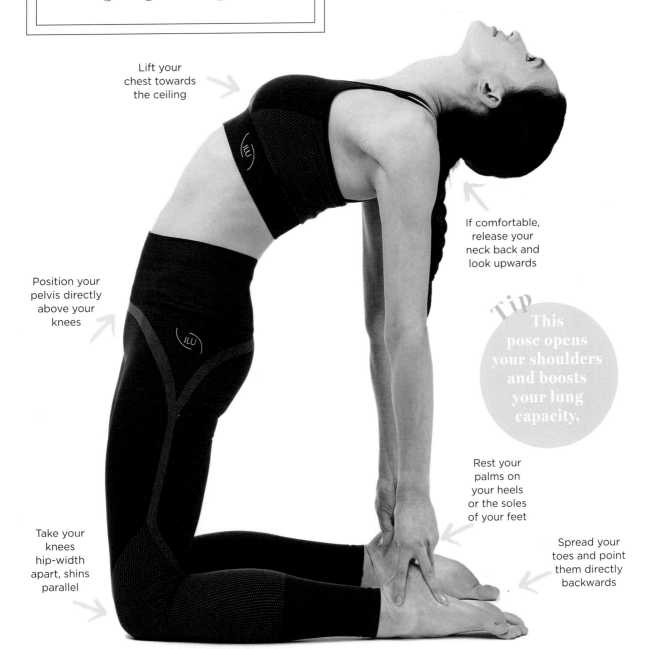

CAMEL
Key alignment points

Lift your chest towards the ceiling

If comfortable, release your neck back and look upwards

Position your pelvis directly above your knees

Tip This pose opens your shoulders and boosts your lung capacity.

Rest your palms on your heels or the soles of your feet

Take your knees hip-width apart, shins parallel

Spread your toes and point them directly backwards

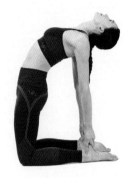

Ustrasana
IN-DEPTH FORM GUIDE

Getting into the pose

● Sit on your heels with your hands resting on your thighs and take a couple of breaths to centre yourself. When you feel ready, kneel up and take your knees hip-width apart, keeping your thighs vertical, shins parallel and the tops of your feet flat on the floor. Spread your toes and point them directly backwards.

● With your pelvis square, in neutral and floating over your knees, lift up from your waist to your chest, creating length in your spine. Open your chest and lengthen evenly through your spine, creating an arc from your pelvis to your neck.

Work in the pose

● Roll your shoulders up, back and down, then reach your hands to your feet, resting your palms on your heels or the soles of your feet. Firm your thighs and root down through your legs, tailbone and arms and feel the corresponding lift in your torso.

● Maintain an even curve the length of your spine and connect to this sense of expanding in two directions – from your waist down through your tailbone, and from your waist up to your chest.

● Draw your collarbones away from each other to open the front of your chest more, keep releasing your shoulder blades down your spine. If comfortable, release your neck backwards and close your eyes. Breathe normally in the pose for as long as is comfortable, for up to half a minute.

> 66 *Connect to a sense of expanding in two directions – waist down through your tailbone and waist up to your chest* 99

Coming out of the pose

● There are a couple of ways you can come out of Camel. Either engage your core, inhale and release your hands as you come up to vertical, or exhale and lower your buttocks onto your knees – this will be easier for your back, but will place more strain on your knees. Experiment with both versions and once you're familiar with how each feels, decide which method to use according to how your body feels in the moment.

● Rest for a few moments in Legs up the wall (p34), then make any notes you wish to about your experience.

Modifications

Inflexible?

Rest on the balls of your foot; place a rolled blanket beneath your ankles; take your hands to blocks either side of your foot; rest the back of your head on a wall; take one hand at a time to your heels.

Hypermobile?

Keep your stretched muscles active – your front thighs, core and upper arms.

Injured?

Neck issues: keep your chin towards your chest. Sensitive knees: place a folded blanket beneath them.

GO DEEPER

1 Keep the front of your throat soft

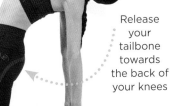

Slide the tips of your shoulder blades down your back and the inner edges towards each other

Release your tailbone towards the back of your knees

Draw your front ribs in to prevent compression in your back

2

Roll your inner thighs back slightly

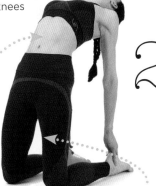

4

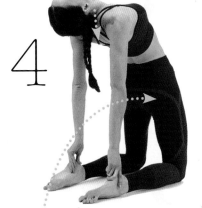

Keep your buttock muscles relaxed

Draw your mid-back towards your front heart

Lengthen your arms from your shoulders to your heels

3

Practice notes   Use this space to deepen your experience of the pose, making notes on any challenges, what felt good and the areas to focus on in the future.

_____

_____

_____

_____

_____

BOW
Dhanurasana

Meaning: dhanu (bow)

Another pose for relieving hunched up shoulders, Bow is also great for strengthening your back muscles and opening your chest and hip flexors – the muscles that become tight from too much sitting. Aim to balance the lift of your legs by actively engaging your upper back muscles.

PREPARATION

✦ Cat/Cow (p30) ✦ Cow face pose (p31) ✦ Crescent moon (p32)

BENEFITS

MUSCLES/JOINTS
✦ Opens your chest
✦ Strengthens your back and legs
✦ Stretches your front body
✦ Tones your abdominals

PHYSIOLOGICAL
✦ Aids your respiration
✦ Boosts your immunity (increases T-cell production)

SUBTLE/THERAPEUTIC
✦ Calming
✦ Helps fatigue
✦ Eases constipation
✦ Mentally stimulating

RISKS/PRECAUTIONS

✦ Lower back issues
✦ knee and shoulder injuries

CONTRAINDICATIONS

✦ Very high/low blood pressure ✦ migraines
✦ hernia ✦ serious back issues

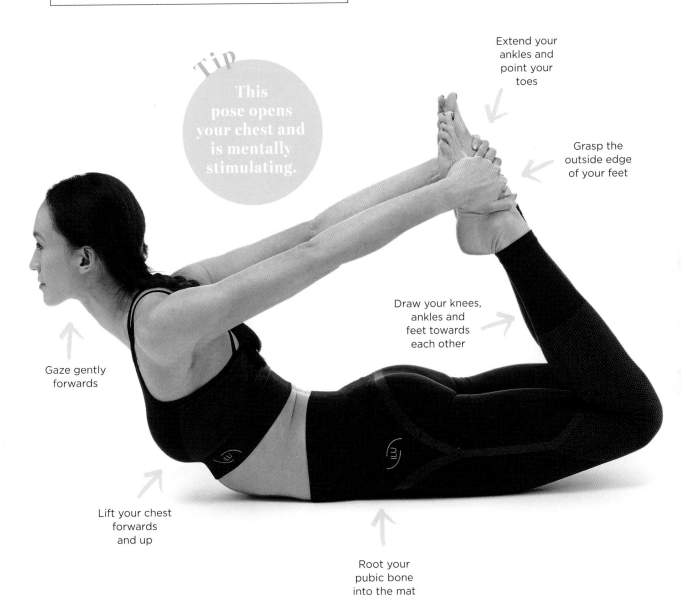

BOW
Key alignment points

Tip

This pose opens your chest and is mentally stimulating.

Extend your ankles and point your toes

Grasp the outside edge of your feet

Draw your knees, ankles and feet towards each other

Gaze gently forwards

Lift your chest forwards and up

Root your pubic bone into the mat

Dhanurasana
IN-DEPTH FORM GUIDE

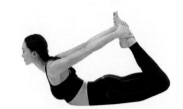

Getting into the pose

● Lie on your stomach with your forehead resting on the floor, arms by your sides, legs straight, feet resting on the tops of your toes. Take a couple of deep breaths to still your mind and become present in your body.

● When you feel ready, rotate your shoulders back down your spine, then bend your knees and reach back to grasp the outside of each ankle with your hands.

● On an inhale, draw your navel in and root your pubic bone into the mat as you lift your chest off the mat. As you exhale, keeping your arms straight, raise your feet upwards and into your hands.

Work in the pose

● Externally rotate your upper arms to open your chest further, and keep drawing your shoulders down your back to create space around your ears. Maintain an even curve throughout the length of your spine. Take a couple of breaths here, then, on an inhale, lift your chest a little higher, pause on the exhale. Repeat once or twice more.

● Breathe deeply and evenly in the pose for up to one minute with your gaze softly forwards. If comfortable, work on bringing your knees, feet and ankles closer together.

Coming out of the pose

● On an exhale, gently release your feet, stretch your legs and lower your arms and legs to the floor and rest your head on one side. If you only stayed up for a few seconds, you can repeat the pose a few times, before coming down to rest in Savasana (p35) and writing up your notes on how felt in the pose.

> ❝ *Maintain an even curve the length of your spine. Take a few breaths, then on inhale, lift your chest a little higher* ❞

Modifications

Inflexible?
Take your knees wider apart; wrap a strap around your feet, one end in each hand; practise raising your chest only, then your feet only.

Hypermobile?
Don't lock your elbow joints; draw your arms into their sockets; focus on lifting your legs rather than arching your spine.

Injured?
Knees: take your knees further apart; flex your feet; spread your toes and reach through the balls of your feet.

GO DEEPER

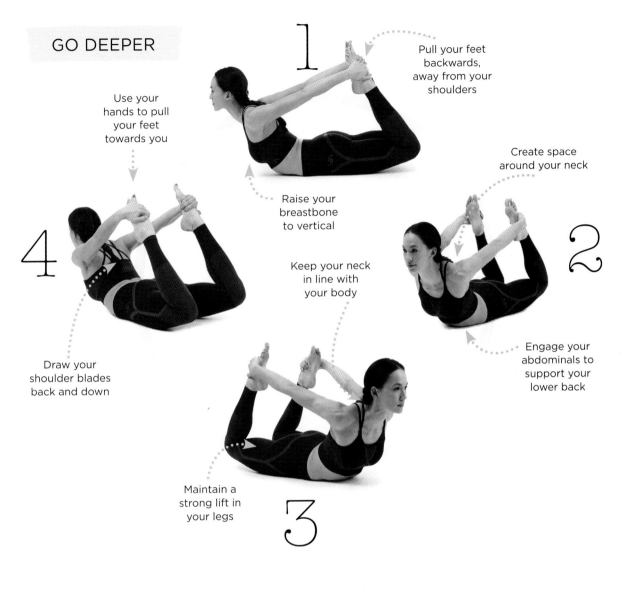

1

Pull your feet backwards, away from your shoulders

Use your hands to pull your feet towards you

Create space around your neck

Raise your breastbone to vertical

Keep your neck in line with your body

4

2

Draw your shoulder blades back and down

Engage your abdominals to support your lower back

Maintain a strong lift in your legs

3

Practice notes   Use this space to deepen your experience of the pose, making notes on any challenges, what felt good and the areas to focus on in the future.

_____

_____

_____

_____

_____

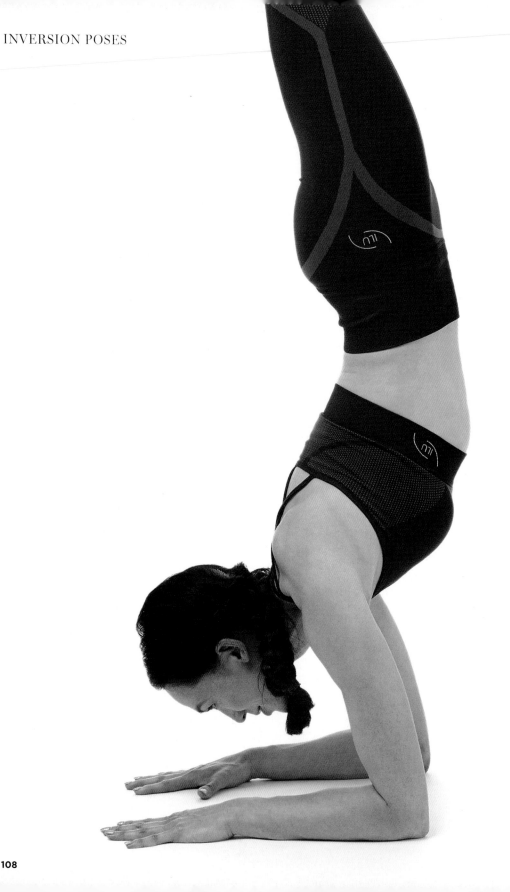

INVERSIONS

When we hear the word inversion, most of us think of *shoulderstand* or headstand, where the body is completely up-side-down. But an inversion is any pose where your *head is below your heart*, so Downward dog and Legs up the wall (p34) also qualify. They have so many benefits, such as *flooding your brain with oxygen*, boosting immunity, enhancing balance and *building up your core strength*, that it's worth taking time with this chapter. In the early days of your period, practise Legs up the wall instead of the stronger inversions – you'll still enjoy some of the benefits of being upside down.

DOWNWARD-FACING DOG
Adho mukha svanasana

Meaning: adho (down), mukha (mouth or face), svana (dog)

Downward dog is a great pose to do when you feel tired, as it quickly energises you and, when practised regularly, rejuvenates your whole body. It's more important to create length in your spine than touching your heels on the floor, so focus initially on lifting your tailbone back and up.

PREPARATION

✦ Cat/Cow (p30) ✦ Thread the needle (p31) ✦ Reclining hand to toe (p32)

BENEFITS

MUSCLES/JOINTS

✦ Strengthens your wrists, hands, arms, shoulders and legs
✦ Stretches your fingers, arms, toes, calves and hamstrings
✦ Opens your hips, elongates and releases tension in the spine
✦ Opens your chest

PHYSIOLOGICAL

✦ Strengthens the nerves in your arms, legs and spine
✦ Rejuvenates your spinal discs

SUBTLE/THERAPEUTIC

✦ Eases stress, mild depression, insomnia and fatigue
✦ Relieves asthma and sinusitis
✦ Helps sciatica and back pain
✦ Relieves hot flushes

RISKS/PRECAUTIONS

✦ Wrists and shoulders ✦ hamstrings
✦ mild high blood pressure ✦ headache ✦ wrist and shoulder issues ✦ disc injury ✦ menstruation

CONTRAINDICATIONS

✦ Carpel tunnel syndrome ✦ high blood pressure
✦ glaucoma ✦ detached retina ✦ diarrhoea

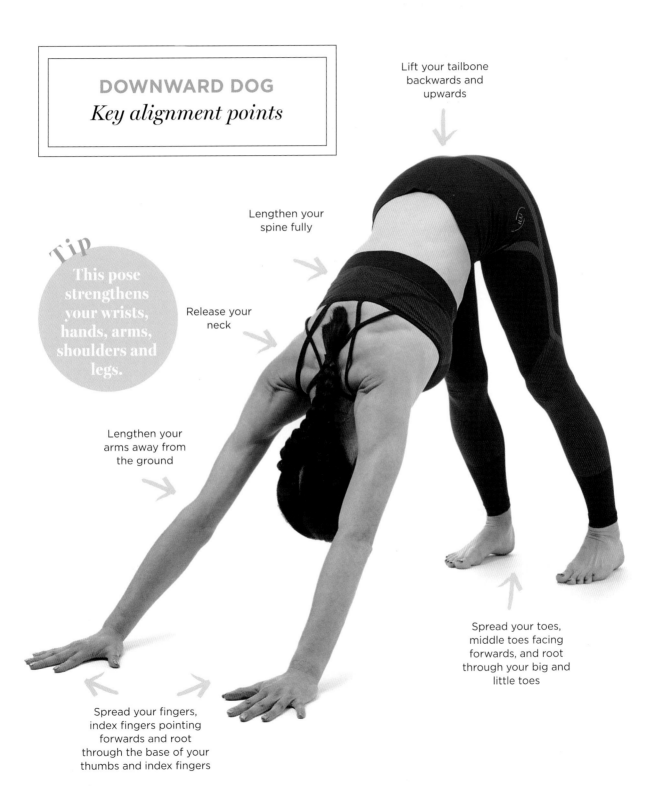

DOWNWARD DOG
Key alignment points

Lift your tailbone backwards and upwards

Lengthen your spine fully

Tip
This pose strengthens your wrists, hands, arms, shoulders and legs.

Release your neck

Lengthen your arms away from the ground

Spread your toes, middle toes facing forwards, and root through your big and little toes

Spread your fingers, index fingers pointing forwards and root through the base of your thumbs and index fingers

Adho mukha svanasana
IN-DEPTH FORM GUIDE

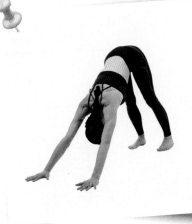

Coming into the pose

● Begin on all-fours, with your hands a palm's length in front of your shoulders, shoulder-width apart, fingers spread and index fingers facing the front of the mat. Have your knees directly beneath your hips and your shins parallel. Tuck under your toes.

● Root through the base of your thumbs and index fingers, then raise your knees off the mat, drawing your tailbone back and up to lengthen your spine.

● Keep your knees bent initially, checking they are in line with your middle toes, and focus on extending your spine by grounding through your hands (imagine you are pushing the floor away from you). Rotate your upper arms externally and draw your shoulder blades down your spine. Lower your front ribs towards your thighs and release your neck.

> " *Notice what you're experiencing in your body. Direct the in-breath to areas of tension, yield into the pose as you exhale* "

Work in the pose

● Take a couple of breaths, then bring your attention to your hips. Take your tailbone further back and up, maintaining a slight backbend in your spine, then gently draw one heel and then the other towards the mat, stretching out your hamstrings in a walking motion.

● Spread your toes and lower both heels. If they reach the ground, check that your weight is evenly distributed through each foot and your inner arches are lifted.

● Breathe, be present. Notice what you're experiencing in your body. Direct the in-breath to any areas of tension, yield into the pose as you exhale. See if you can radiate two lines of energy from your navel, one down your arms and through the centre of your palms and the other from your navel down your legs and through the soles of your feet.

● Be here for up to one minute savouring the sensations you are feeling.

Coming out of the pose

● When you feel ready, exhale, gently lower your knees and go into Child's pose – sitting back on your heels, torso resting on your thighs and arms at the sides of your body, palms by your hips. Then rest in Savasana (p35) for a few minutes before reflecting on how your body feels now, and making any notes about your experience.

Modifications

Inflexible?
Raise your heels; bend your legs; take your feet wider apart; bend and straighten your legs alternately; rest your hands hip-height on a wall, arms and torso horizontal, legs vertical.

Hypermobile?
Don't lock your knees; keep your arms active, extended away from the floor; engage your core to support your spine.

Injured?
Wrists: rest on your fists or forearms. Shoulders: turn your fingertips out to the sides or put your hands against a wall. Neck: take your hands wider apart.

GO DEEPER

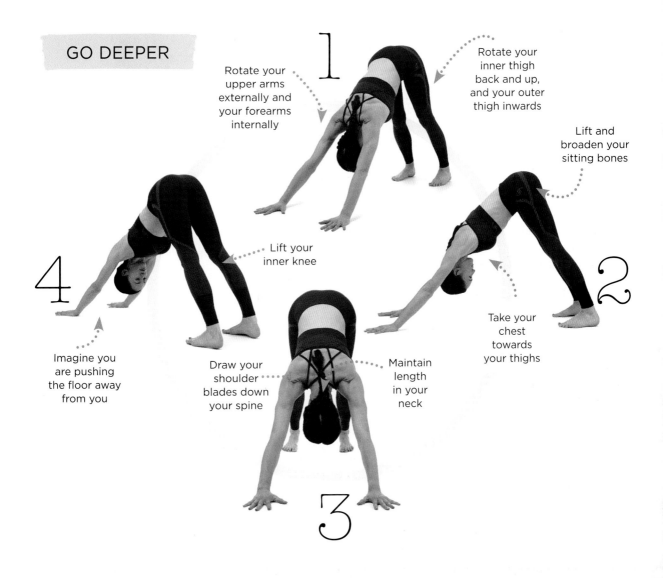

1

Rotate your upper arms externally and your forearms internally

Rotate your inner thigh back and up, and your outer thigh inwards

Lift and broaden your sitting bones

Lift your inner knee

2

Take your chest towards your thighs

4

Imagine you are pushing the floor away from you

Draw your shoulder blades down your spine

Maintain length in your neck

3

Practice notes   Use this space to deepen your experience of the pose, making notes on any challenges, what felt good and the areas to focus on in the future.

SHOULDERSTAND
Salamba sarvangasana

Meaning: salamba (propped up), sarvanga (all the limbs of the body)

Known as the queen of yoga poses, Shoulderstand is said to integrate your mind, body and soul, according to BSK Iyengar. If you're new to the pose, protect your neck by placing two folded blankets on the floor. Place your shoulders three inches from the edge and rest your head on the floor.

PREPARATION

✦ Cat/Cow (p30) ✦ Cow face pose (p31) ✦ Bicycle twist (p33)

BENEFITS

MUSCLES/JOINTS
✦ Strengthens your arms, legs and spine
✦ Tones your core
✦ Eases tension in your shoulders and neck
✦ Firms your buttocks

PHYSIOLOGICAL
✦ Increases blood flow to your brain
✦ Stimulates your thyroid gland

SUBTLE/THERAPEUTIC
✦ Reduces stress and fatigue
✦ Eases insomnia
✦ Relieves menopause symptoms
✦ Improves your digestion

RISKS/PRECAUTIONS

✦ Neck pain ✦ headache
✦ low blood pressure

CONTRAINDICATIONS

✦ Neck or back injury ✦ diarrhoea ✦ menstruation
✦ high blood pressure

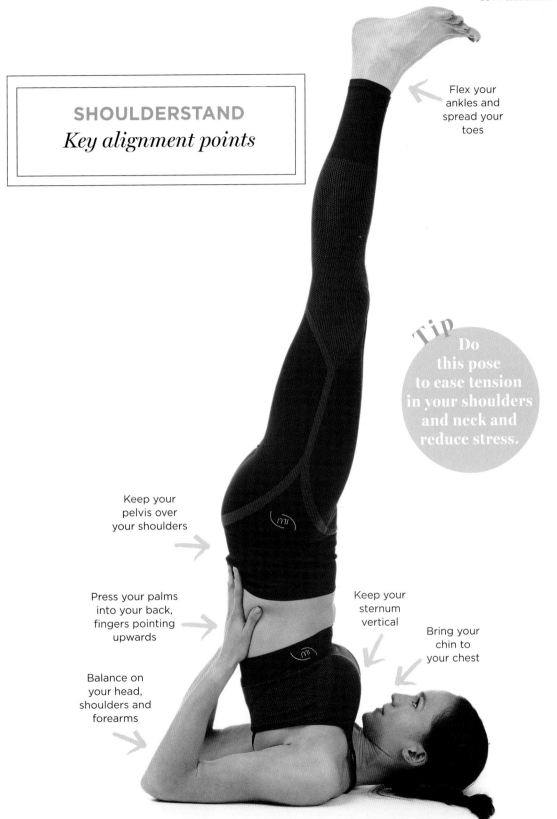

SHOULDERSTAND
Key alignment points

Flex your ankles and spread your toes

Tip
Do this pose to ease tension in your shoulders and neck and reduce stress.

Keep your pelvis over your shoulders

Press your palms into your back, fingers pointing upwards

Keep your sternum vertical

Bring your chin to your chest

Balance on your head, shoulders and forearms

Salamba sarvangasana
IN-DEPTH FORM GUIDE

Getting into the pose

● Lie on your back with your knees bent, feet flat on the floor and arms out to the sides, palms facing upwards. Take three deep breaths into your belly to release any tension. When you feel ready to begin, exhale as you raise your sacrum to bring your knees over your chest.

● Inhale, then exhale and root through your elbows to raise your torso, lifting your buttocks to the ceiling and your knees towards your head. Place your palms on your back to support your spine.

● Snuggle your shoulders towards each other and draw your elbows close to your body. On an exhale, roll back a little further to take your hips directly over your shoulders and slowly raise your feet towards the ceiling. Press your hands into your back to help bring your spine into vertical, and reach up strongly, lengthening your inner and outer legs upwards, so your body is perpendicular to the floor from your shoulders to your toes.

Work in the pose

● Lift through the balls of your big toes, lengthening your inner legs. Draw your shoulder blades down your spine and in towards your heart. Lift your sternum to vertical.

● Root through your shoulders and upper arms and feel the corresponding lift in your torso.

● Draw the sides of your waist horizontally towards your centre, and your upper and lower abdomen vertically towards your navel. This will support your spine and help maintain the lift in your torso and legs.

● Beginners can stay in the pose for 10 to 20 breaths, breathing slowly and evenly into your belly. Gradually build up to five minutes as your strength improves.

Coming out of the pose

● On an exhale, bend your knees in to your chest, release your arms and slowly uncurl your spine to release down to the floor, one vertebra at a time. Rest in Savasana (p35) for five minutes, then make any notes you wish to.

> " *Beginners can stay in the pose for 10 to 20 breaths, breathing slowing and evenly into your belly* "

Modifications

Inflexible?
Practise with your back facing a wall; do half Shoulderstand, with your torso at 45 degrees to the floor and hips bent to 90 degrees.

Hypermobile?
Engage your core; micro-bend your knees.

Injured?
Neck issues: rest your shoulders on three folded blankets. Back issues: practise against a wall.

GO DEEPER

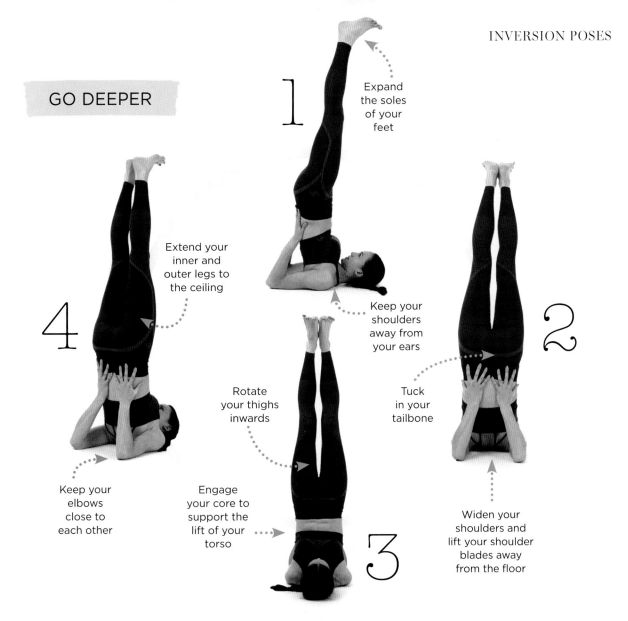

1 — Expand the soles of your feet

Keep your shoulders away from your ears

Tuck in your tailbone

2 — Widen your shoulders and lift your shoulder blades away from the floor

Rotate your thighs inwards

Engage your core to support the lift of your torso

3

Extend your inner and outer legs to the ceiling

4 — Keep your elbows close to each other

Practice note — Use this space to deepen your experience of the pose, making notes on any challenges, what felt good and the areas to focus on in the future.

_____

_____

_____

_____

_____

SUPPORTED HEADSTAND
Salamba sirsasana

Meaning: salamba (supported), sirsa (head)

Headstand is one of the most important asanas, which is why it's often referred to as the king of yoga poses. By flooding the brain with fresh oxygen and nutrients, it rejuvenates your entire system. To balance the pose, always do Shoulderstand (p114), either before or after Headstand.

PREPARATION

✦ Cow face (p30) ✦ Boat (p33) ✦ Plank (p33)

BENEFITS

MUSCLES/JOINTS
✦ Strengthens your arms and shoulders
✦ Creates space between your vertebra
✦ Tones your core and back
✦ Strengthens your inner thighs

PHYSIOLOGICAL
✦ Drains lymph fluid from your legs
✦ Balances your nervous and endocrine systems

SUBTLE/THERAPEUTIC
✦ Improves your digestion
✦ Boosts the circulation to your brain
✦ Calming and energising
✦ Enhances your pituitary function

RISKS/PRECAUTIONS

✦ Low blood pressure ✦ menstruation

CONTRAINDICATIONS

✦ High blood pressure ✦ back and neck injuries
✦ glaucoma ✦ migraine ✦ shoulder issues

SUPPORTED HEADSTAND
Key alignment points

Flex your heels and spread your toes

Align your knees and feet over your pelvis

Align your pelvis over your shoulders

Draw your navel to your spine

Tip
This pose strengthens your arms and shoulders and is calming.

Interlace your fingers and cup your head in your hands

Keep your elbows shoulder-width apart

Salamba sirsasana
IN-DEPTH FORM GUIDE

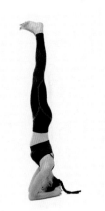

Getting into the pose

● Begin on all-fours and lower your forearms to the floor, elbows shoulder-distance apart. Clasp your hands together with your fingers interlaced and thumbs resting on your index fingers and then rest your hands on your little finger edge. If you find it more comfortable, tuck in the little finger that touches the floor so it rests next to the little finger on the other hand.

● Lean forwards and rest the front of the crown of your head on the floor and cup your head with your hands. Keep your neck long and your shoulders away from your ears. Straighten your legs, lifting your buttocks and rest on the tips of your toes. Slowly edge your toes forwards as far as you can while keeping your legs straight.

● When your hips are over your shoulders, engage your core, bend your knees and lift them to your chest, so that you're in a reverse tuck position, torso vertical, knees pointing down and toes pointing to the ceiling.

● Keep contracting your core as you slowly extend your legs straight upwards, ankles flexed.

Work in the pose

● Keep rooting through your forearms and wrists – this not only protects your neck from compression and potential injury, it also helps you lift your torso.

● Engage your core to support your lower back, and lift strongly through your inner and outer legs, using ujjayi breathing (p23).

● Initially, remain in the pose for 10 to 20 breaths, and gradually increase the time you spend in the pose to 10 minutes, using the 'Go deeper' tips on the facing page to help your refine your alignment.

Coming out of the pose

● On an exhale, slowly and with control, come out of the pose in the way you went in – lowering into a reverse tuck, then walking your feet away from your head. Rest for a moment in Child's pose – sitting back on your heels, torso resting on your thighs and arms at the sides of your body, palms by your hips. Lie in Savasana (p35), for five minutes, then write up your practice notes.

> 66 *Engage your core to support your lower back, and lift strongly through your inner and outer legs* 99

Modifications

Inflexible?
Practise in the corner of a room where two walls meet at right angles, and rest your feet on the wall.

Hypermobile?
Fully engage your arms, shoulders, core and legs; micro-bend your knees.

Injured?
Low blood pressure: come out of the pose slowly. Menstruation: only stay in the pose a short time.

GO DEEPER

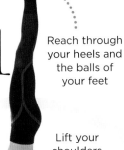

1 Reach through your heels and the balls of your feet

Lift your shoulders up away from the floor

Stretch the backs of your knees and your thighs

4 Hug your shoulder blades in to your spine

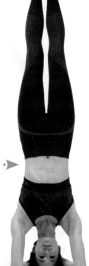

2 Align your elbows with your shoulders

Draw the sides of your waist and your upper and lower abdominals towards your navel

Squeeze your inner thighs and hug your legs in to the mid-line

Send your energy downwards from your waist, and upwards through your legs

3

Practice notes   Use this space to deepen your experience of the pose, making notes on any challenges, what felt good and the areas to focus on in the future.

_____

_____

_____

_____

_____

FOREARM BALANCE
(FEATHERED PEACOCK POSE)

Pincha mayurasana

Meaning: pincha (feather) mayura (peacock)

It looks challenging, but if you can do Headstand (p118), you'll soon be proficient in Pincha. The strength you built up in Headstand, particularly by pressing your forearms into the ground, is crucial to this pose. You can also prepare for it with core work, such as Plank and Boat poses (p33).

PREPARATION

✦ Cow face pose (p31) ✦ Crescent moon (p32) ✦ Plank (p33)

BENEFITS

MUSCLES/JOINTS
✦ Strengthens your arms, shoulders and back
✦ Tones your abdominals
✦ Stretches your neck, shoulders and chest
✦ Strengthens your wrists

PHYSIOLOGICAL
✦ Boosts your energy
✦ Increases blood flow to your abdominal organs

SUBTLE/THERAPEUTIC
✦ Calms your brain
✦ Aids your digestion
✦ Eases mild depression
✦ Improves your balance

RISKS/PRECAUTIONS

✦ Low-blood pressure
✦ menstruation

CONTRAINDICATIONS

✦ Elbow, neck and back injuries ✦ high blood pressure ✦ glaucoma ✦ migraine ✦ shoulder issues

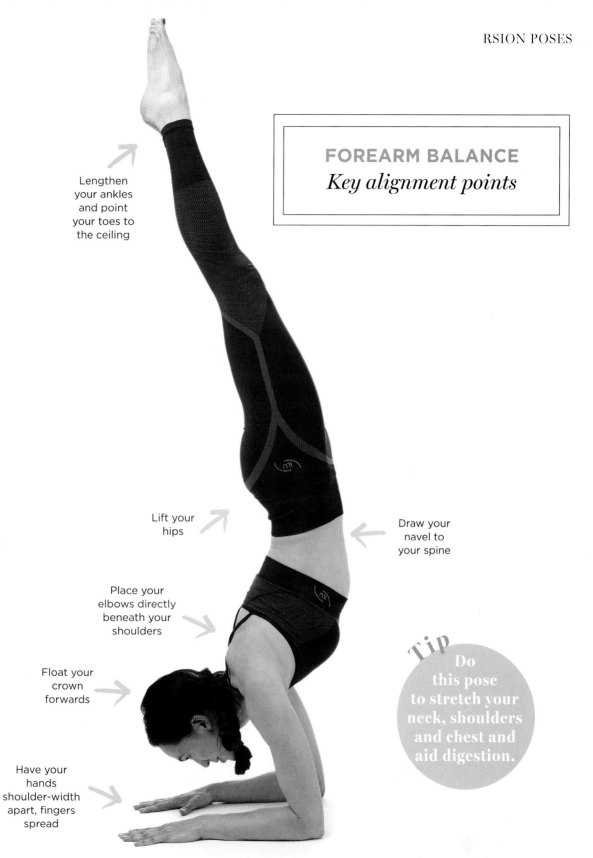

Lengthen
your ankles
and point
your toes to
the ceiling

FOREARM BALANCE
Key alignment points

Lift your
hips

Draw your
navel to
your spine

Place your
elbows directly
beneath your
shoulders

Tip

Do
this pose
to stretch your
neck, shoulders
and chest and
aid digestion.

Float your
crown
forwards

Have your
hands
shoulder-width
apart, fingers
spread

Pincha mayurasana
IN-DEPTH FORM GUIDE

Getting into the pose
● Begin in a modified Downward dog pose (p112) with your forearms on the floor, elbows directly beneath your shoulders and forearms parallel. Position yourself so that your fingers are almost touching the skirting board. Establish a strong foundation by spreading your fingers, rooting through your inner wrists and the base of your thumbs and index fingers, and press the centre of your forearms into the mat.
● Bend one leg and balance on the ball of this foot. Work the foot towards your chest, keeping your other leg straight. Take a few small hops, exhaling each time, to swing your straight leg upwards. With each hop, lift your straight leg a little higher. Eventually you'll reach a height where your bent leg will naturally lift off the floor too. You'll need to use enough momentum to take your hips over your shoulders. Initially, your heels may hit the wall forcefully, but over time, and with repeated practice you'll develop more control. Remember to swap over your leading leg each time you practise Pincha, so you don't create an imbalance in your muscles.

Work in the pose
● Draw your navel to your spine to support your lower back, and strongly engage your legs, lifting from your tailbone through to your toes.
● Ensuring your forearms are vertical, draw your shoulder blades away from each other and your front ribs inwards.
● When you first begin working with Feathered peacock, it may be enough to stay in the pose for just five or 10 breaths, but as you become more stable, you can work towards staying in the pose for up to a minute. Let experience guide you.

Coming out of the pose
● On an exhale, and maintaining the lift in your shoulders, lower one leg at a time with control. Rest in Savasana (p35) for as long as you need then, if you wish to, make notes on your experience for the next time you practise the pose.

" As you become more stable, you can work towards staying in the pose for up to a minute. Let experience guide you "

Modifications

Inflexible/beginner?
Place a block between your hands, shoulder-width apart. Do modified Downward dog facing away from the wall, at a distance so you can walk your feet up the wall, taking your legs parallel to the floor.

Hypermobile?
Lift strongly out of your shoulders; engage the core; put a strap round your upper arms.

Injured?
Low-blood pressure: practise for a short time; come out of the pose slowly. Menstruation: don't practise the pose during the first few days of your period and don't stay long in the pose.

GO DEEPER

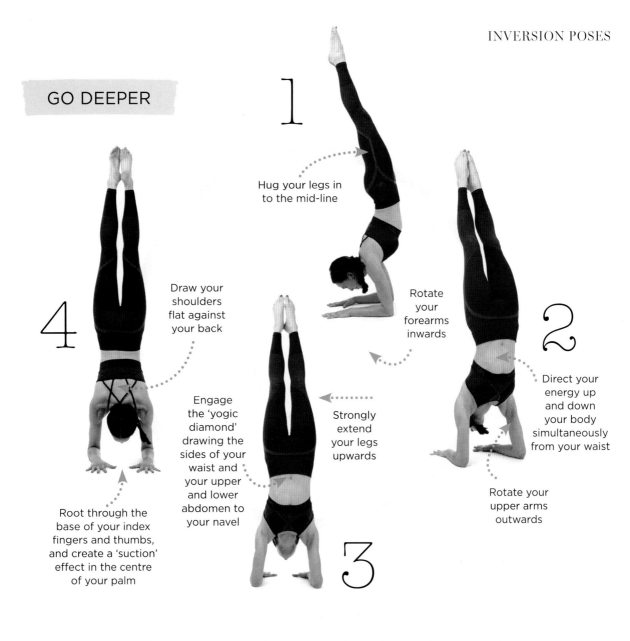

1

Hug your legs in to the mid-line

Rotate your forearms inwards

Draw your shoulders flat against your back

4

Engage the 'yogic diamond' drawing the sides of your waist and your upper and lower abdomen to your navel

Strongly extend your legs upwards

2

Direct your energy up and down your body simultaneously from your waist

Rotate your upper arms outwards

Root through the base of your index fingers and thumbs, and create a 'suction' effect in the centre of your palm

3

Practice notes   Use this space to deepen your experience of the pose, making notes on any challenges, what felt good and the areas to focus on in the future.

_____

_____

_____

_____

_____

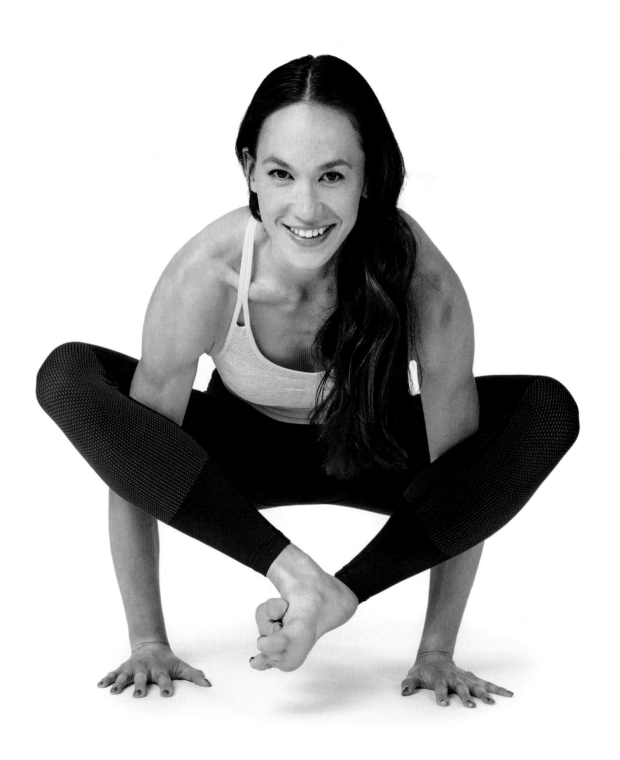

DIRECTORY

Apparel

ACTIVE IN STYLE
activeinstyle.com

ASQUITH
asquithlondon.com

EVERY SECOND COUNTS
everysecondcounts.co.uk

FROMYOGA
fromclothing.com

ILU
ilufitwear.com

LULULEMON
lululemon.co.uk

MADEBYYOGIS
yogaclicks.store

MANDUKA
manduka.com

M LIFE
mlifelonfon.com

NOBALLS
noballs.co.uk

PURE LIME
purelimeshop.com

STYLE PB
stylepb.com

SWEATY BETTY
sweatybetty.com

UNDER THE SAME SUN
underthesamesun.se

WELLICIOUS
wellicious.com

Equipment

EKOTEX YOGA
ekotexyoga.co.uk

GAIAM
gaiam.co.uk

HOLISTIC SILK
holisticsilk.com

MADEBYYOGIS
yogaclicks.store

MANDUKA
manduka.com

YOGA BLISS
yogabliss.co.uk

YOGA MATTERS
yogamatters.com

YOGA STUDIO
yogastudio.co.uk

DIRECTORY

Find a teacher

THE BRITISH WHEEL OF YOGA
bwy.org.uk

YOGA ALLIANCE
yogaalliance.co.uk

JUDITH HANSON LASATER
judithhansonlasater.com

SARAH POWERS
sarahpowers.com

SHIVA REA
shivarea.com

TRIYOGA
triyoga.co.uk

YOGA WITH SIMON LOW
simonlow.com

Online yoga classes

EKART YOGA
ekhartyoga.com

MOVEMENT FOR MODERN LIFE
movementformodernlife.com

GAIA
gaia.com

YOGAGLO
yogaglo.com

YOGAIA
yogaia.com

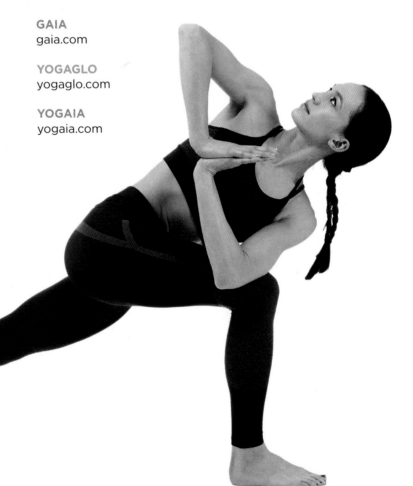

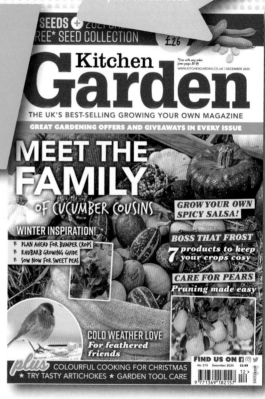
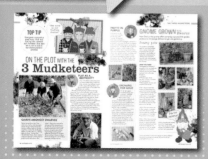
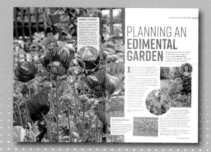
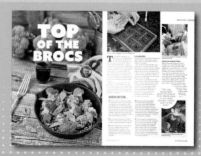

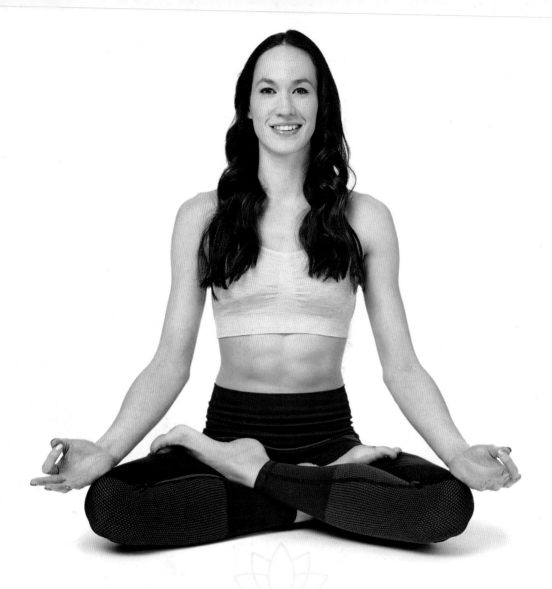

FAREWELL

Congratulations on working your way through this guide. We hope you've begun to enjoy some of the benefits of workshopping individual yoga poses and seen improvements to your overall practice as well. You'll probably have noticed that many of the alignment cues are transferable to other poses – grounding through your feet, supporting your lower back with your core, expanding your energy out through your centre. As you develop your ability to deeply tune in to your body and mind, you'll soon find that you naturally apply what you've learnt here to other postures, guiding your practice in the way that is right for you. In yoga, as in life, if you stay present, stay open and listen to your innate wisdom, the rest will naturally unfold. Be well.

Eve